To Pit

Clinical Neuropharmacology

MONOGRAPHS IN CLINICAL PHARMACOLOGY
Volume 4

General Editor
Daniel L. Azarnoff M.D.
Senior Vice President
Worldwide Research and Development
G. D. Searle & Co.
Chicago, Illinois
Formerly Professor of Medicine and Pharmacology
University of Kansas

ALREADY PUBLISHED

Clinical Pharmacology of Psychotherapeutic Drugs   Leo E. Hollister M.D.
Drugs and Renal Disease   William M. Bennett M.D.
Drug Treatment of Gastrointestinal Disorders   Norton J. Greenberger M.D.,
   Constanti Arvanitakis M.D., and Aryeh Hurwitz M.D.

FORTHCOMING VOLUMES IN THE SERIES

Pediatric Clinical Pharmacology   Lars O. Boreus M.D.
Clinical Pharmacology in Pulmonary Disease   R. B. Cole M.D., F.R.C.P.
Clinical Cardiovascular Pharmacology   David Shand M.B., Ph.D.
Drugs for Rheumatic Disease   Carl M. Pearson M.D., Harold Paulus M.D. and
   Daniel Furst M.D.

Clinical Neuropharmacology

HENN KUTT, M.D.

Associate Professor, Departments of Neurology and Pharmacology
Cornell University Medical College
New York, New York

FLETCHER MCDOWELL, M.D.

Professor of Neurology, Associate Dean
Cornell University Medical College
New York, New York
Director, Burke Rehabilitation Center
White Plains, New York

with a contribution by

HENRY MASUR, M.D.

Assistant Professor of Medicine, Divisions of
Infectious Diseases and International Medicine
Cornell University Medical College
New York, New York

and

HENRY W. MURRAY, M.D.

Assistant Professor of Medicine, Divisions of
Infectious Diseases and International Medicine
Cornell University Medical College
New York, New York

CHURCHILL LIVINGSTONE
New York   Edinburgh   London   1979

© Churchill Livingstone Inc. 1979

Distributed in the United Kingdom by Churchill Livingstone, Robert Stevenson House, 1-3 Baxter's Place, Leith Walk, Edinburgh EH1 3AF and by associated companies, branches and representatives throughout the world.

First published 1979
Printed in USA
ISBN 0 443 08009 7

Library of Congress Cataloging in Publication Data

Kutt, Henn.
  Clinical neuropharmacology.

  (Monographs in clinical pharmacology; v. 4)
  Bibliography: p.
  Includes index.
  1. Nervous system—Diseases—Chemotherapy.
2. Neuropharmacology. I. McDowell, Fletcher Hughes,
joint author. II. Title. III. Series. [DNLM:
1. Nervous system diseases—Drug therapy. W1
M0567KP v. 4 / WL100.3 C641]
RC350.C54K87   616.8'04'61   79-19226
ISBN 0-443-08009-7

General Editor's Foreword

I remember as a medical student my wonder about the prespicacity of neurologists in the pinpointing of lesions within the central nervous system. Gradually, however, I came to realize that although making the correct diagnosis is a satisfying intellectual exercise and the basis of all therapy, it is of less value if physicians are unable to satisfactorily cure or even ameliorate the associated disorders. I also soon learned there was only minimally effective therapy for the majority of neurological disorders. There is still a long way to go, and the problem is compounded by the lack of regenerative capacity of some nervous tissue components, but significant progress has been made in understanding the pathophysiology of and in developing effective therapy for neurological disorders. An up-to-date accounting of our present knowledge will be found in this monograph.

The first and last chapters deserve special mention. The Introduction, in addition to providing an overview of the current status of treatment of disorders of the nervous system, contains a useful discussion of the general principles and factors affecting drug usage. More and more drugs are being found to have a significant adverse effect on the nervous system. These drugs and the mechanisms involved are discussed in the last chapter along with suggestions for preventing or treating the reactions.

This monograph contains several features that are useful for the practicing physician. For example, for each antiepileptic drug, the factor needed to calculate the conversion of plasma drug levels from μg/ml to μM is given. In the quest for international standardization, the latter unit (not frequently used in the United States) will be seen in the literature more and more.

This monograph will provide therapeutic information for the neurologist as well as the physician involved in general health care delivery. I recommend it to you.

Daniel L. Azarnoff, M.D.

Preface

This book is intended to be of use to students in health fields as well as to physicians concerned with the treatment of disorders of the nervous system. It points out that the physician has perhaps as much to offer in the treatment of neurologic disorders as he does in the treatment of cardiac, renal or endocrinologic disorders. Many of the disorders of the nervous system are chronic conditions requiring continuous supplementative medication which ameliorates but does not cure the disease. The margin between an effective and a toxic dose of medication is often narrow, and considerable expertise and laboratory support may be required in regulating the dosage. There is considerable need for more effective neuropharmacologic treatment with the development of new drugs, new approaches, and new knowledge regarding the pathophysiology of disorders of the nervous system. While waiting for this to develop, the application of the growing knowledge of pharmacokinetic and pharmacodynamic aspects of the available drugs used in the treatment of neurologic disorders, based on monitoring of drug blood levels, has improved the efficacy of therapy of some conditions such as seizure disorders, Parkinson's disease, and nervous system infections. Similar improved efficacy is likely to occur in the treatment of myasthenia gravis, migraine, and movement disorders, as practical methodology for monitoring the concentrations of drugs develops and the empirical data base for effective and toxic drug concentrations accumulates. These aspects of treatment are emphasized in this book along with a warning that, due to variations in the severity of the disease process and acquired tolerance, the effective and toxic drug doses and blood level concentrations vary among individual patients. Thus, in making the clinical decision regarding drug dosage, both clinical findings and laboratory data need to be considered carefully.

Much of what is included in this book is based on personal experience and reflects particular points of view. This, however, is integrated with information and data compiled from the literature listed in the bibliography as well as with that derived from the experience and opinions of our colleagues.

For the physician concerned with the treatment of neurologic disorders, this book should be considered only as a base to enlarge his understanding of treatment through careful attention to the ever expanding neuropharmacologic field and new possibilities for treatment.

Henn Kutt, M.D.
Fletcher McDowell, M.D.

Contents

1. INTRODUCTION — 1

2. SEIZURE DISORDERS — 12

3. EXTRAPYRAMIDAL SYNDROMES — 54

4. CEREBROVASCULAR DISEASES — 76

5. MYASTHENIA GRAVIS (M.G.) — 92

6. MULTIPLE SCLEROSIS — 101

7. HEAD PAIN — 106

8. NERVOUS SYSTEM COMPLICATIONS WITH SYSTEMIC METABOLIC DISORDERS — 114

9. VITAMIN DEFICIENCIES   **127**

10. TREATMENT OF MALIGNANT GLIOMAS   **133**

11. INFECTIONS OF THE NERVOUS SYSTEM • Henry Masur, M.D.,
and Henry W. Murray, M.D.   **136**

12. DRUG-INDUCED DISORDERS OF THE NERVOUS SYSTEM   **189**

1

Introduction

Disorders of the nervous system may result from an abnormal process or state in the nervous system itself, or may reflect the response of the nervous system to some systemic abnormal processes. Often, the precise mechanism leading to the disorder is not known, and treatment consists of alleviation of the most disturbing symptoms. There are few disorders in which one course of treatment alone eradicates the cause, thus resulting in cure. The underlying abnormal state or process in many disorders is long lasting once it has developed, and may require prolonged and continuous suppressive or supplementary therapy. In still other disorders, drug therapy may have no effect at all on the cause of the disorder and its symptoms. Thus, effective treatment of neurological disorders with drugs is limited to a relatively few disease entities.

Complete cure may be achieved in some nervous system infections using antimicrobial agents, if therapy is started in time and extensive structural damage to the nervous system has not occurred. Cures can also be achieved with vitamins in some nutritional or metabolic neuropathies and encephalopathies, if the therapy is started before irreversible changes have taken place. The key here is early treatment, because of the poor regenerative potential of the nervous tissues. Therefore the emphasis should be on preventive, more than on curative programs.

Dramatic symptomatic relief can be achieved with drug therapy in several disorders of the nervous system. These include seizure disorders, extrapyramidal syndromes, facial pain and migraine headaches, as well as myasthenia gravis and some spastic states. With the exception of migraine, the relief of symptoms in these disorders requires continuous administration of drugs over long periods of time. The drugs are usually needed until spontaneous remission of the disease process occurs; or sometimes, for the rest of the patient's life.

Drug treatment is modestly effective in cerebrovascular disease, where it may alleviate the outcome or diminish the occurrence of vascular occlusions to some extent in some patients. In multiple sclerosis, drug therapy can beneficially influence the course of an acute exacerbation but has little, if any effect on the long-term, general course of the disease. Recent advances in the chemotherapy of malignant brain tumors are encouraging, but at best can only prolong the survival time by a modest degree.

The course of degenerative and/or hereditary diseases such as amyotrophic lateral sclerosis, Friedreichs' ataxia, olivo-ponto-cerebellar degeneration and muscular dystrophies, has remained virtually unaffected by any of the currently available chemotherapeutic agents.

This somewhat pessimistic picture may improve as continuing research efforts clarify the mechanisms of the disease processes and develop new therapeutic agents.

GENERAL PRINCIPLES OF TREATMENT

Pharmacodynamic Aspects

The pharmacodynamic aspects deal with the biological effects of the drug, including the therapeutic and the toxic effects.[16] In the laboratory, under experimental conditions one can accurately establish the minimal effective dose of the drug and show an increasing therapeutic effect with increasing the dose, as well as define the toxic range of the dose. The dose-response principle holds true in clinical situations in general. It would be desirable to be able to carry out pharmacodynamic measurements, i.e., to quantitate the severity of the disease process and the therapeutic and toxic effects of drugs in patients. This would allow valid comparison of the existing effective drugs and be useful in the development of new drugs. Numerical values of drug effects can be obtained in some clinical situations such as prothrombin time with anticoagulants. More often than not, however, measuring the therapeutic and toxic effects in patients, poses various problems. Thus, an epileptic patient may not remember all the generalized tonic-clonic seizures he has had; and the observer may lose count of the absence episodes. Prolonged electroencephalographic recording and telemetry will provide accurate seizure counts, but due to the complexity of the apparatus, are not generally applicable yet. It is also not easy to accurately quantitate the clinical manifestations of intoxication due to high doses of some drugs such as anticonvulsants. Here, one may use numerical grades on, for instance, a scale of 0 to 5 in estimating the severity of sedation or equilibrium disturbances.

With some drugs, the therapeutic and toxic effects correlate to some extent with the concentration of the drug in the blood.[2,9,14] Thus, the blood levels can be used as rough guidelines in evaluation of the pharmacodynamic parameters. One must realize, however, that the severity of the disease process varies among individual patients, as does the tolerance to intoxication. Therefore, a universally applicable therapeutic dose and blood concentration for a drug is not expected.[14]

The aim in the therapy is to match the severity of the disease with a dose that renders effective drug concentrations. In patients with very severe disease process, this may require doses and concentrations which cause intoxication or other intolerable side effects. A compromise dosage that produces the greatest benefit and the least intoxication or side effects may have to be settled for in these patients. Adjusting the dose to achieve effective concentration of the drug is facilitated by knowledge about some aspects of the pharmacokinetics of the drug.

Pharmacokinetic Aspects

Pharmacokinetic aspects deal with the fate of a drug in the organism and are reflected mainly by the measurements of concentrations of the drug (and its metabolites) in the available body fluids and tissues.[3,6,16] Knowledge of the fate of the drug is helpful in obtaining the best possible therapeutic effect with an agent. The pharmacokinetic aspects relevant in treatment are (1) absorption (indicating how soon to expect the effect), (2) elimination (indicating how long the effect may last), and (3) distribution (indicating when and how much of the drug might reach the desired location).

Absorption   There are two major concerns regarding drug absorption: (1) the time at which the peak blood level occurs following oral ingestion and (2) the total amount absorbed from a dose. A rapid absorption peak is desirable with analgesics and antimigraine drugs. Incomplete absorption may necessitate parenteral administration.[3,6]

Many drugs used in the treatment of disorders of the nervous system are well absorbed. These include most of the antiepileptic drugs, cholinergic drugs and antimicrobial agents. Anticholinesterases, on the other hand, are incompletely absorbed, and the oral dose greatly exceeds the parenteral dose.

The rate and completeness of absorption generally depends upon the physical-chemical properties of a drug such as solubility, ionization and particle size.[3,16,21] Furthermore, the absorption of a drug can be enhanced or inhibited by the previous or simultaneous ingestion of other substances. For instance, the absorption of ergotamine is enhanced by caffeine. The absorption of phenytoin, on the other hand, may be inhibited by simultaneously ingested antacids; thus, a treatment failure with an otherwise effective agent can result from poor absorption in an individual patient, a situation which can be remedied by removing the inhibiting agent. Taking drugs with meals generally does not reduce the total amount absorbed, but tends to delay the absorption peak.

Elimination   The rate and mechanism of the elimination of a drug depends basically upon its physical-chemical properties. Many drugs must undergo extensive and nearly complete biotransformation before they can be eliminated, while others are excreted unchanged in large amounts.[3,4] The rate of elimination of the active drug determines the duration of the effect of a single dose and influences the extent of accumulation of the drug in the body during chronic administration. The elimination rate to some extent parallels the plasma half-life.

The plasma *half-life* is defined as the time it takes for the plasma level to decline 50 percent from a previous value.[16,21] That decline is usually exponential. Drugs with a short half-life such as anticholinesterases need to be given frequently, if continuous, effective concentration is to be maintained. Several antiepileptic drugs have long half-lives and can be given once a day. Following the onset of chronic administration of drugs, there is a rise of drug concentration in the body over a period of days, until the intake and output are in balance and a plateau or steady state is achieved. Only then can one expect to see the maximum effect of a given dose. Empirically, it has been proven that the time it takes to reach the steady state or maximum concentration with a given dose is 4 to 6 times the half-life. Thus, if the half-life of phenobarbital is approximately 3 days, the achievement of steady state takes over 2 weeks. Although the half-life of a drug in the majority of patients falls into a definable range of values, it is important to know that variations among individuals can be considerable; and that the half-life of a drug can change with age[20] in the same individual. The half-life and the rate of elimination of a drug can be influenced by a variety of factors. Thus, alkalinization enhances the elimination of phenobarbital, while phenobarbital, in turn, can enhance the elimination of other drugs by inducing enzymes that are involved in their biotransformation.

Biotransformation of drugs usually effects an increase in the solubility of the drug, thus preparing it for elimination.[4,16] Frequently occurring metabolic steps include hydroxylation, followed by conjugation with glucuronic acid or sulfate. In this process, the drug also becomes inactivated. Drugs that carry alkyl radicals such as methyl are usually first dealkylated. The des-methyl or ''nor'' intermediary metabolites are usually pharmacologically active until they are further metabolized and eliminated.

The biotransformation of drugs is carried out largely in the liver by the microsomal enzyme system. The rate of activity of these enzymes is determined in part by genetic make-up of the patient, but it can also be influenced by environmental factors. Among the environmental factors of clinical significance are other drugs that can either enhance or inhibit the enzymes involved in the biotransformation of the primary drug. These drug-drug interactions at the drug biotransformation stage are seen with some antiepileptic drugs[12] and with coumarine anticoagulants[19] leading to a change in the half-life and the rate of elimination, and consequently to a change in dosage requirement.

Distribution   After absorption the drugs distribute from the blood into the tissues according to their ability to penetrate the various compartments and the existing drug concentration gradients.[16,18] Active transport mechanisms through the cell membranes may be involved in the distribution of some drugs. With the majority of drugs used in the treatment of nervous system disorders, it is important that they can penetrate into the nervous tissue. The ability to pass the blood-brain barrier depends upon the physical-chemical properties of the drug and generally increases with increasing lipid solubility of the agents. Most antiepileptic drugs reach the brain easily in concentrations equal to concentrations in the blood or higher. The speed of entry, however, varies among drugs. For instance, diazepam concentration in the brain reaches maximum within 5 minutes after intravenous injection, that of phenytoin takes 10 to 20 minutes, while phenobarbital concentration reaches maximum in about 30 minutes. This is relevant when treating status epilepticus with phenobarbital in that repeating the phenobarbital dose too soon because of lack of rapid action, may, eventually, result in overdosing. Many antimicrobial agents, on the other hand, pass the blood-brain barrier or spinal fluid barrier modestly or poorly, although that passage may be enhanced considerably by inflammation. Those antimicrobial agents that penetrate poorly, even in the presence of inflammation, need to be given intrathecally or intraventricularly (if they are the only agents to which the infecting organism happens to be sensitive).

Low ability to enter the central nervous system may also be an advantage. Such is the case with some anticholinesterases. They can be given to patients with myasthenia gravis in large amounts without causing central nervous system related side effects.

Penetration of levodopa into the brain is modest, and necessitates a relatively high dose and blood concentration to achieve therapeutic effect. This creates a problem because the peripheral dopa decarboxylase then produces large amounts of dopamine outside the nervous system which leads to systemic side effects such as vomiting and hypotension. The situation can be alleviated, fortunately, by using dopa decarboxylase inhibitors which do not enter the brain, thus preventing excessive systemic dopamine formation.

Plasma protein binding has some effect on drug distribution. Many drugs are bound to plasma proteins, mostly albumin, to a greater or lesser extent.[8,10] For instance, of the total phenytoin concentration in plasma, 90 percent is bound. This leaves 10 percent free to penetrate into the tissues. A decrease of phenytoin binding to 80 percent, as is often seen in patients with chronic uremia or liver disease,[17] doubles the amount of free drug to enter the brain. The clinical corollary to that is, that often in uremic patients very low total plasma phenytoin concentrations may be effective.

Pharmacogenetic Aspects

Pharmacogenetic factors are relevant in drug therapy of nervous system disorders mainly by their influence upon the activity of enzymes involved in the biotransformation of some drugs.[1,7,22,23] For instance, there is a (rarely occurring) familial incidence of individuals who can metabolize and eliminate only small amounts, (100 to 200 mg), of phenytoin per day. The common dose of 300 mg daily constitutes an overdose to those slow phenytoin metabolizers, and leads to severe drug accumulation and intoxication. Conversely, other individuals may metabolize phenytoin rapidly and thus require higher than average doses to maintain average effective drug concentrations in the blood.[11]

The genetic make-up of a patient can influence his response to phenytoin indirectly, via his phenotype regarding isoniazid inactivation. Isoniazid strongly inhibits phenytoin biotransformation. Its concentration with the common clinical doses, however, in moderate and fast isoniazid inactivators remains too low to have a significant effect upon phenytoin biotransformation. In the very slow isoniazid inactivators, on the other hand, concentrations of active isoniazid that are sufficient to cause marked phenytoin accumulation and intoxication can be present. Thus an epileptic, who is otherwise an average phenytoin metabolizer, becomes a slow phenytoin metabolizer if he acquires tuberculosis, is given isoniazid, and happens to be a very slow isoniazid inactivator. His phenytoin dose then needs to be adjusted downward accordingly.[13] The slow isoniazid inactivator is also liable to other complications related to isoniazid per se, such as peripheral neuropathy and hepatitis.[7]

Another (rarely occurring) genetic anomaly is associated with abnormal pseudocholinesterase. Patients thus inflicted have an exaggerated response to succinylcholine when, for instance, treated with this agent for tetanus.[15]

There is some evidence that the degree by which hepatic drug metabolizing enzymes can be induced by the "inducer" drugs is influenced by the genetic factors.[24,25] It has been demonstrated that the degree of acceleration of aminopyrine metabolism by phenobarbital is identical in identical twins but may vary considerably in non-identical twins. Based on clinical observations, it appears that the phenobarbital effect upon the biotransformation and elimination of other drugs also varies considerably among individuals. Addition of phenobarbital may cause a considerable decline of phenytoin blood level in some rare patients but may have little, if any, effect in the majority.[11,12] It may increase the requirement of coumarine anticoagulant dosage in some patients and have little effect in others. It is fair to assume that these individual differences are at least in part influenced by the genetic make-up of the patients.

BLOOD LEVELS

Clinical experience has shown that monitoring of drug blood levels can be useful for obtaining the optimal therapeutic success. This is particularly true with those drugs that need to be given continuously to control symptoms of an established disease process.[2,9,14,26] The usefulness of application of drug blood levels in the clinical management of patients has evolved and gained recognition during the past decade and a half. This has prompted increasing numbers of clinical laboratories to set up capability for performing these assays. There are currently available, assays of many drugs that produce concentrations in the blood in the microgram per milliliter range. Availability of blood levels of drugs found in nanograms or picograms per milliliter is still limited.

Of the drugs used for the treatment of nervous system disorders, blood level determinations are now generally available for most major antiepileptic drugs and some analgesics, antimicrobial agents and vitamins. Less readily available at the present time are measurements of ergot preparations, anticholinesterases and levodopa. The reliability of these assay values depends upon the methods used and the experience and the strictness of the quality control of the laboratory.

The rationale of the application of blood levels in clinical management is based on the following empirical findings.

(1) Pharmacokinetic findings: There is a reasonably good correlation between the dose and the blood level of many drugs in most individual patients. When the dose is increased, the blood level rises fairly proportionately until the dose becomes high enough to saturate the elimination mechanism; then a disproportional upswing of blood level occurs. The same dose does not usually produce the same blood level in all individuals. The differences in blood levels with the same dose may reflect individual differences in absorption, biotransformation and/or elimination, and may be caused by genetic or environmental factors. There is, however, a definable range of blood levels from a given dose. Defining the range of blood levels to be expected in the majority of patients with a dose is clinically useful. If the observed blood level value in a particular patient is well below or above the level range expected from his dose, one may

suspect noncompliance, drug-drug interactions, or some unusual individual pharmacokinetic peculiarity.[14]

(2) Pharmacodynamic findings: The blood levels correlate to some extent with the clinical effects of the drug. As the level increases, amelioration of symptoms continues but very high levels are usually associated with intoxication or dose related side effects. If blood levels of a large enough population have been studied, often a range of levels can be defined above which optimal effectiveness is observed in the majority of patients. Similarly, with some drugs a level range can be defined above which the intoxication or predictable side effects are expected to occur in the majority of patients.[2,9,14] These ranges must make allowances for the variations in the severity of the disease process and variations in the individual tolerance to the drug. All taken into consideration, the expected, effective and potentially toxic blood level ranges are clinically useful. A low level explains inadequate clinical response; a level in the usually effective range with inadequate therapeutic response indicates above average severity of the disease process, or wrong drug; and a high blood level range in the presence of dose-related side effects confirms intoxication.

The two key questions then to be asked when utilizing blood levels in clinical management are: (1) Is the observed blood level within the range that is expected from the prescribed dose? (2) Is the observed blood level commensurate with the clinical response? The answers to these questions can be analyzed by considering the pharmacokinetic and pharmacodynamic findings described in the two preceding paragraphs.

Since the expected blood level ranges from a dose, the effective level ranges, and the potentially toxic blood level ranges are empirically derived from clinical observations, they cannot be used as rigid criteria. They are to be used as general guidelines together with a thorough clinical evaluation of the patient in making clinical decisions. If used with that in mind, the blood level data can greatly contribute to the successful management of the patient.

INTERACTIONS BETWEEN DRUGS

Numerous interactions between concurrently administered drugs are known to occur.[5,12,16] Some of these reactions are interesting biochemical phenomena without any clinical consequences, while others may influence the therapeutic effects or may cause intoxication. Some interactions are invoked knowingly by prescribing a second drug which will enhance the therapeutic effect and/or decrease the toxic effects of the primary drug. Other interactions may be clinically useful if small, but harmful if large in magnitude. Finally, some drug interactions may occur in a few apparently unusually susceptible patients, while the majority of patients can take the same drug combination without difficulties. The phrase "drug-drug interaction" is mostly used in association with those interactions that cause or have the potential to cause undesired clinical effects.

There are a variety of mechanisms involved in the interactions between drugs. They can occur in the process of drug absorption, biotransformation and elimination, distribution or at the site of action.

Drug absorption from the intestinal tract can be influenced by another drug either by increasing or decreasing the gastrointestinal mobility. Another mechanism involved in absorption is alteration of solubility of one drug by the other. In some instances the particular incipient used by some manufacturers of tablets or capsules has reduced the solubility and absorption of the active ingredient.

The *interaction involving drug biotransformation* and elimination comes about primarily by means of two mechanisms. The first is inhibition of biotransformation of one drug by the other. The inhibition may be the result of the second drug competing for the enzymes involved in the biotransformation of the primary drug.[12] It may also result from noncompetitive inhibition if the other drug has an enzyme inhibiting effect (e.g., disulfiram). Whether the inhibition is competitive or noncompetitive, the result is accumulation of the primary drug which, if extensive, leads to intoxication.[11] When the inhibiting drug cannot be discontinued for clinical reasons, the dose of the primary drug is reduced and a new dose titrated with the help of blood level determinations, if available.[12] It is a common occurrence that a drug which causes clinically significant inhibition of biotransformation of the primary drug in some patients has little if any effect in others. Reasons for this variation in the response are not all clear. One mechanism that has been observed is that the affected patient is a slow metabolizer of the inhibiting drug.[13] An unusually vulnerable enzyme system and defective co-factor pool are other possibilities to be considered.

The second mechanism of interaction at the biotransformation stage is enzyme induction. A well-known inducer of hepatic microsomal enzymes is phenobarbital, but other antiepileptic drugs can also induce these enzymes. If the inducing drug is metabolized by the same enzymes, thus competing with the primary drug, the net effect may be negligible as is often the case.[12] Furthermore, as already alluded to in the section on pharmacogenetics, the extent of enzyme induction varies among individuals.[23,24,25] Therefore, the clinically significant consequences of enzyme induction are not as frequent as one might expect on theoretical grounds. They seem to occur in some susceptible individuals or with particular drugs.

Interactions involving the drug distribution occur when one drug affects the active transport mechanism of the other.[5,16] Another mechanism in this category is competition for the binding sites of plasma proteins between the primary and the interacting drug. The displacement of the primary drug with resulting increase in the unbound fraction of the primary drug has played a clinically significant role with anticoagulants.

Interactions may occur at the site of action.[5,16] Thus diazepam increases some central effects of methadone without significantly raising its blood level. A more clearly understood interaction at the site of action may occur in antimicrobial therapy. An agent that stops the multiplication of microorganisms diminishes the effects of an agent that is effective during cell division. Conversely, a synergistic action is obtained in antitumor therapy by selecting agents that act by different mechanisms.

The clinically relevant specific interactions with drugs used in the treatment of nervous system disorders are discussed in sections with these drugs.

REFERENCES

1. ASBERG M, EVANS DAP, SJOKVIST F: Genetic control of nortriptyline in man. J Med Genet 8:129–135, 1971.
2. EADIE MJ: Plasma level monitoring of anticonvulsants. Clin Pharmacol 1: 52–66, 1976.
3. FINGL E: Principles of drug absorption, distribution and metabolism. In: Antiepileptic Drugs: Quantitative analysis and interpretation. (eds): CE Pippenger, JK Penry, H Kutt. Raven Press, New York, pp 221–236, 1978.
4. GLAZKO J: Antiepileptic drugs: Biotransformation, metabolism and serum half-life. Epilepsia 16: 367–391, 1975.
5. GRAHAME-SMITH DG: Drug interactions. University Park Press, Baltimore, 1977.
6. GREENBLATT DJ, KOCH-WESER RJ: Clinical Pharmacokinetics. N Engl J Med 293: 702–705, 964–970, 1975.
7. HUGHES HB, BIEHL J, JONES AP et al: Metabolism of isoniazid in man as related to the occurrence of peripheral neuritis. Am Rev Tuberc 70: 266–273, 1954.
8. JUSKO WJ, GRETCH M: Plasma and tissue protein binding of drugs in pharmacokinetics. Drug Met Rev 5: 43–140, 1976.
9. KOCH-WESER J: Serum drug concentrations as therapeutic guide. N Engl J Med 287: 227–231, 1972.
10. KOCH-WESER J, SELLERS EM: Binding of drugs to serum albumin. N Engl J Med 294: 311–316, 526–531, 1976.
11. KUTT H: Biochemical and genetic factors regulating Dilantin metabolism in man. Ann N Y Acad Sci 179: 704–722, 1971.
12. KUTT H: Interactions of antiepileptic drugs. Epilepsia 16: 393–402, 1975.
13. KUTT H, BRENNAN R, DEHEJIA H, et al: Diphenylhydantoin intoxication. A complication of isoniazid therapy. Amer Rev Resp Dis 101: 377–384, 1970.
14. KUTT H, PENRY JK: Usefulness of blood levels of antiepileptic drugs. Arch Neurol 31: 283–288, 1974.

15. LaDu B: Plasma esterase activity and the metabolism of drugs with ester groups. Ann N Y Acad Sci 179: 684–693, 1971.
16. Melmon KL, Morelli HF: Clinical Pharmacology. MacMillan Co, N. Y., 1978.
17. Odar-Cederlof J, Borga O: Kinetics of diphenylhydantoin in uremic patients: consequences of decreased plasma protein binding. Eur J Clin Pharmacol 7: 31–37, 1974.
18. Oldendorf WH: Blood-brain barrier permeability to drugs. Ann Rev Pharmacol 14: 239–248, 1974.
19. O'Reilly RA: The pharmacodynamics of the oral anticoagulant drugs. Prog Hemostasis Thromb 2: 175–213, 1974.
20. Rane A, Wilson JT: Clinical pharmacokinetics in infants and children. Clin Pharmacokinet 1: 2–24, 1976.
21. Smolen VF: Theoretical and computational basis for drug bioavailability determinations using pharmacological data. II Drug input response relationships. J Pharmacokinet Biopharm 4: 355–375, 1976.
22. Vesell ES: Application of pharmacokinetic principles to the elucidation of polygenically controlled differences in drug response. J Pharmacokinet Biopharmac 1: 521–540, 1973.
23. Vesell ES: Pharmacogenetics. Biochem Pharmacol 24: 445–450, 1975.
24. Vesell ES, Page JG: Genetic control of the phenobarbital-induced shortening of plasma antipyrine half-lives in man. J Clin Invest 48: 2202–2209, 1969.
25. Vesell ES, Passananti GT, Greene FE, Page JG: Genetic control of drug levels and of the induction of drug-metabolizing enzymes in man: Individual variability in the extent of allopurinal and nortriptyline inhibition of drug metabolism. Ann N. Y. Acad Sci 179: 752–773, 1971.
26. Walle T, Conradi EC, Walle UK, et al: The predictable relationship between levels and dose during chronic propranolol therapy. Clin Pharmacol Ther 24: 668–677, 1978.

2

Seizure Disorders

Paroxysmal events characterized by convulsive movements and/or altered states of consciousness may result from a variety of reasons. Some of them are related to systemic abnormalities such as hypoglycemia, hypocalcemia, pyridoxine deficiency and some toxic states. When the underlying mechanism in such instances is recognized and appropriately treated, the seizures abate. In a narrower sense, the patients diagnosed as having seizure disorders either fall into the category of epilepsy of unknown origin, or of epilepsy secondary to some known predisposing factor that usually has caused damage to brain tissue.

PREDISPOSING FACTORS

Head and Brain Injury

Head trauma is among the most common of factors leading to seizure disorders in young adult patients. Following a severe closed head injury, about 5 percent of patients develop residual seizures within a year or two. Following head injuries with penetration of skull and dura, up to 50 percent of patients develop seizure disorders within several months or a year or two.[21] Injury to the brain can also occur during birth, due to compression in the birth canal.

Brain Tumor

Brain tumors are found in 10–15 percent of patients who start having nonfocal, generalized seizures at the age of early adulthood or in later years. In the presence of focal seizures, the incidence of brain tumors is higher. In children the majority of brain tumors occur in the subtentorial region and do not cause seizures.[35,63]

Infections

Acute infections such as meningitis, encephalitis and brain abscess are often associated with seizures. These infections can also cause damage to the brain that results in chronic seizure disorder.

Cerebrovascular Disease

Arteriosclerotic disease with or without occlusion of a major cerebral vessel is often present in patients who start having seizures after the age of 50. Cerebral aneurysm, arteriovenous malformations and collagen diseases with brain vessel involvement are other vascular diseases which may be associated with seizure disorders.

Genetic Factors

The role of genetic factors in the genesis of seizure disorders is not clear. The chances of a child developing seizure disorder are somewhat greater, if one of the parents had a primary generalized seizure disorder (absence or tonic-clonic) and are even greater if both parents are so afflicted. Yet, what is transmitted genetically is probably the disposition to seizures rather than the manifest seizure disorder. It is thought that the offspring of epileptic parents may develop a seizure disorder from a lesser environmental cause than the offspring of nonepileptic parents.[41]

In many patients with seizure disorders no known predisposing factor is present and the disorder in these instances is classified as idiopathic epilepsy or seizure disorder of unknown origin.

SEIZURE PROCESS

The basic abnormality in the seizure disorder is still largely obscure. Although the predisposing factors discussed above often result in damaged areas or scars in the brain, not all scars cause seizures. It may be then assumed that the damage involves a critical area and must be in just the right proportion in order to create an epileptic focus. Electrophysiologic studies have shown that in the vicinity of the focus are abnormal nerve cells, the epileptic neurons,[57,68,69] that emit bursts of high frequency discharges. These at times build to a continuous high frequency (up to 1000 per second) activity, leading eventually to propagation to adjacent areas and clinical seizure manifestations.[68] The glial cells surrounding the epileptic neurons may be abnormal as well, in that they have lost their ability to maintain the normal potassium gradients.[76] The spread of seizure discharge probably utilizes post-tetanic potentiation along its path. The extent of spread determines whether a partial focal seizure or a generalized seizure occurs. It may be assumed that epileptic neurons also exist in some unknown area in patients with idiopathic epilepsy manifested by primary generalized seizures. What leads the epileptic neuron to abnormal discharging is not clear. It is best to assume at this time that it is based on some deranged biochemical process. It may also be assumed that the severity of that process varies among individuals, since some patients have rarely occurring seizures which are easily suppressed by antiepileptic drugs, while others have frequent seizures which are more difficult to suppress.[28,38]

SEIZURE TYPES

The clinical manifestations of seizures depend, in part, upon what area of the brain they originate from, in part upon what pathways are involved in the spread of seizure discharges, and in part upon the patient's age. Seizures originating from deep subcortical structures tend to manifest as generalized tonic-clonic seizures in adults, while in young children with less mature brains, absence seizures occur more commonly. When the seizures originate from cortical or near cortical foci, the manifestations start as partial focal seizures, which may or may not spread and become generalized.

SEIZURE CLASSIFICATION

The nomenclature of seizures has undergone considerable change in the past decade. The terms which have traditionally been used; grand mal, petit mal, minor motor, focal and psychomotor epilepsies, are being replaced by terms that allow for more precise definitions of those seizure types. It appears now, that since the publication of the *International League Against Epilepsy Classification of Seizures* nearly a decade ago,[13] its terminology is being used more and more often in communications and texts dealing with epilepsy. The main advantage of the nomenclature of the *International Classification* is that it enables different observers to come to the same conclusions regarding the seizure types better than the previously used terminologies. The clinical relevance of proper seizure classification lies in the observation that some seizure types respond best to treatment with certain drugs.

The *International Classification* primarily considers the site of origin of the seizure and the extent of spread of seizure activity. There are four groups of seizures; (1) generalized seizures, (2) partial seizures, (3) unilateral seizures, and (4) unclassified seizures (see Table 2-l).[9,13]

Generalized Seizures

This group contains eight subcategories and includes manifestations in which activation of widespread areas of brain occurs suddenly. The activation usually originates from the deep subcortical structures. Among the predominant generalized seizure types are the following:

Generalized tonic-clonic seizures with sudden loss of consciousness, followed first by stiffening, then bilateral jerking movements and finally by postictal stupor. These seizure types correspond to the traditional grand mal seizures.

Absence seizures either simple or complex. This category comes nearest to the traditional definition of pure petit mal seizures. The patient stops whatever

---

Table 2-1 / International League Against Epilepsy Classification of Seizures

I. Partial seizures (begin locally) with elementary symptomatology (usually without impairment of consciousness)
        With motor symptoms
        With sensory or somato-sensory symptoms
        With autonomic symptoms
        Compound forms
  Partial seizures with complex symptomatology (usually with impairment of consciousness)
        With cognitive symptomatology
        With affective symptomatology
        With psychosensory symptomatology
        With psychomotor symptomatology
        Compound forms
  Partial seizures secondarily generalized
II. Generalized seizures (bilaterally symmetrical and without local onset)
        Absence (petit mal), simple or complex
        Bilateral massive epileptic myoclonus
        Infantile spasms
        Clonic seizures
        Tonic-clonic seizures (grand mal)
        Atonic seizures
        Akinetic seizures
        Tonic seizures
III. Unilateral seizures (or predominantly)
IV. Unclassified epileptic seizures (due to incomplete data)

Adapted from Gastaut H: Clinical and electroencephalographic classification of epileptic seizures. Epilepsia 11: 102–113, 1970

activity he is engaged in, is out of contact, stares or blinks briefly and exhibits little or no other motor manifestations. There are generalized, 3-per-second spike-and-wave bursts in the electroencephalogram during the episode.

Myoclonic and akinetic attacks with brief, prominent jerking movements or sudden loss of muscle tone and falling. In previous terminologies, these seizures were included in the category of "minor motor." Generalized slow spike-and-wave bursts occur in the electroencephalogram.

Infantile spasms with the clinically characteristic nodding movements, and the high voltage irregular slow wave activity in the electroencephalogram (hypsarrhythmia).

Partial Seizures

Partial seizures are often associated with acquired focal lesions in the brain located in or near the cerebral cortex. The electroencephalogram may show focal abnormal discharges. The major subcategories in this group are the following:

Partial seizures with elementary symptomatology either motor, sensory or automatic. This group includes limited focal seizures without loss of consciousness.

Partial seizures with complex symptomatology which involve impairment of consciousness and disturbance of cognitive, affective and psychomotor or psychosensory functions. These manifestations were mostly categorized as psychomotor and temporal lobe epilepsies in the traditional terminology.

Partial seizures, secondary generalized These seizure types correspond to the grand mal seizures with focal onset as defined by traditional terminology.

Unilateral Seizures

This is a group of rarely occurring manifestations where the epileptic discharges appear predominantly over one of the hemispheres.

Unclassified Seizures

This is a group which includes those seizures that do not fit into any other group. It also serves as a provisional classification until further observations and studies reveal additional information which may allow reclassification within groups one through three.

Patients often have several types of seizures, thus termed, mixed seizure disorder.

ANTIEPILEPTIC DRUGS

The established and currently used antiepileptic drugs belong to the following chemical groups: hydantoins, barbiturates, succinimides, oxazolidinediones, benzodiazepines and 5H-dibenzo(b.f.)azepine. These drugs possess a heterocyclic nucleus and are fairly lipid soluble.[28,74] The newcomer valproate is a branched fatty acid. All are eliminated slowly, which allows maintenance of relatively stable concentrations in the body during chronic administration. Some (primidone, trimethadione) are converted into active metabolites which also accumulate in the body. Finally, none of the currently available antiepileptic agents cures epilepsy. They simply suppress the epileptic process and prevent the spread of seizure discharges.

Historical Notes

A large number of agents has been used to treat epileptic patients. A reviewer in late 19th century concluded that there is hardly a substance that at one time or another has not been used against epilepsy and thought to have been effective. Herbs and simple inorganic compounds, including sulfuric acid had been used in medieval times. In the early part of 19th century, salts of iron, iodine, zinc, and silver as well as digitalis, belladonna, opium, mistletoe, and oil of wintergreen were among the agents prescribed to epileptic patients.

The discovery of the first effective agent, potassium bromide, came about in 1857, from the assumption that epilepsy was caused by masturbation, and bromide was known to suppress libido. Following that, bromide was used extensively. It was calculated that at the end of 19th century 2.5 tons of bromides were dispensed annually in National Hospital in London.

Discovery of the next effective antiepileptic agent, phenobarbital, came about in 1912, also by chance. It was given as a sedative to patients including epileptics, who then started to have fewer seizures than before. Phenobarbital rapidly became popular because it provided better seizure control with fewer side effects than bromide.

The discovery of phenytoin in 1937 resulted from a systematic laboratory search for agents with antiepileptic properties. The hydantoins were included in that search because of the similarity in their structure to phenobarbital. Phenytoin proved to be clinically effective against generalized tonic-clonic and most partial seizures with little, if any, sedative effect.

A more recent addition to drugs effective against generalized tonic-clonic and partial seizures is primidone. Favorable reports about its effectiveness have appeared since 1952.

The latest addition, effective against generalized tonic-clonic and in particular against partial seizures, that has gained wide clinical acceptance is carbamazepine, an analogue of tricyclic antidepressants. Favorable reports about its effectiveness have appeared since 1962.

The first drug with apparent specificity against absence seizures was trimethadione. Successful clinical trials were reported in 1945. Due to relatively high toxicity of trimethadione, the search continued and led to succinimides. Favorable trials with ethosuximide as an antiabsence agent have been reported since 1951. The latest in line of the antiabsence drugs is valproate, which has gained clinical acceptance since late nineteen-sixties.

Benzodiazepines have also established a position among antiepileptic drugs. Since 1965, diazepam has become the drug of choice in the treatment of status epilepticus. Clonazepam, in use since early nineteen seventies, has proven to have a wide spectrum of effectiveness but is mainly used for treatment of various forms of childhood seizures.[28]

Carbamazepine

Chemical name: 5H-dibenz(b,f)-azepine-5-carboxamide.

Proprietary names: Tegretol, Amizepin, Finlepsin, Neurotol, Stazepin, among others

Molecular weight: 236.26

Factor   to convert concentration from µg/ml to µM is 4.23

Solubility in water: insoluble

Formulation and Indications   Carbamazepine is a relative newcomer among the antiepileptic drugs. It is marketed in tablet form (200 mg). Liquid oral and parenteral forms are not available at this time.

Clinically, carbamazepine is effective against partial complex seizures and also against generalized tonic-clonic and other partial seizures. Another domain for its use is in the treatment of trigeminal neuralgia.

Beneficial psychotropic effects have been observed by some authors and not by others. The theoretical ground for a psychotropic effect lies in the similarity of its chemical structure to tricyclic psychotropic drugs.[7]

Mechanism of Action   Carbamazepine, like phenytoin, suppresses post-tetanic potentiation and modifies synaptic transmission to some extent. It di- *

minishes the afterdischarges, primarily in subcortical areas. The net effect is essentially the prevention of the spread of paroxysmal discharges.[14,22]

Pharmacokinetic Parameters   Absorption of carbamazepine from the intestinal tract is not complete; about 20 percent of the dose appears in the feces. The peak plasma level appears within 4 to 12 hours following ingestion. It is extensively metabolized and 7 or 8 metabolites are recovered in the urine. Of importance is a circulating active metabolite: the 10,11-epoxide of carbamazepine.[12] Carbamazepine induces its own metabolism, as evidenced by some decline of the plasma level and shortening of its plasma half-life during chronic administration. The plasma half-life in patients not previously exposed to carbamazepine is 20 to 40 hours; following months of chronic administration, this may become 15 to 25 hours. The half-life of 10,11-epoxide is shorter than that of the parent compound. Plasma protein binding of carbamazepine is about 80 percent; that of the 10,11-epoxy metabolite about 50 percent.[12,18]

Administration and Blood Levels   Carbamazepine is used either as a single drug or as an add-on medication. The effective doses usually range from 600 to 1200 mg (10–20 mg/kg) per day given in 2 or 3 installments. The dose may be built up within a week or two, if tolerated. The initial side effects are drowsiness and sometimes headache, which usually abate.

Diurnal variations of carbamazepine blood levels occur but they are not marked. The maximum blood level from a given dose is reached in 4 to 6 days. The blood level of the 10,11-epoxide is usually 20–40 percent that of the parent compound, and lower when phenytoin or phenobarbital are also used. Blood levels usually seen with daily doses of 400 to 800 mg range from 2 to 6 μg/ml, with 600 to 1000 mg the range is 4 to 10 μg/ml, and with 800 to 1600 mg it is 6 to 14 μg/ml. Higher doses often do not produce proportionally higher blood levels, in part because of incomplete absorption, and in part because of auto-induction of biotransformation. Clinically effective blood levels range from 5 to 12 μg/ml; higher levels may be associated with evidence of intoxication.[19,30]

Interactions   Carbamazepine metabolism is enhanced by phenytoin and phenobarbital.[4] In return, carbamazepine may enhance phenytoin, clonazepam and warfarin metabolism. These effects are usually of modest extent.[34,56]

Side Effects   Side effects related to high dose and blood levels are nystagmus, ataxia, drowsiness, and sometimes headache. These tend to appear when blood levels exceed 12 μg/ml, but may appear with lower values, particularly when the patient is receiving high doses of drugs producing similar side effects, such as phenytoin.[19,30]

Other side effects of concern are skin rashes (relatively common) and depression of the hematopoietic system in which leukopenia and thrombocytopenia are of the most concern. The leukopenia may occur early as a transient manifestation; a rapid fall of platelet count is an indication for discontinuation of the drug. Liver function disturbance has been observed and a few liver-related fatalities reported.

Carbamazepine in Pregnancy The general experience with carbamazepine in pregnancy is still relatively limited. It appears, though, that the incidence of birth defects in babies born to mothers taking carbamazepine is not greater, and perhaps even smaller, than that caused by other drugs.

Clonazepam

Chemical name: 5-(2-chlorophenyl)-1,3-dihydro-7-nitro-2H-1,4-benzodiazepine-2-one

Proprietary names: Clonopin, Iktoril, Ravitrol, Rivotrol

Molecular weight: 315.7

Factor to convert concentration from ng/ml to nM is 3.17

Solubility in water: insoluble

Formulation and Indications Clonazepam is marketed as tablets of 0.5, 1.0 and 2.0 mg. Parenteral preparations are available in some countries. It is mostly used for the treatment of myoclonic and absence seizures and infantile spasms.

Mechanism of Action The mechanism of action of clonazepam is probably similar to that of diazepam.[14,48]

Pharmacokinetic Parameters Clonazepam is absorbed relatively quickly and completely from the intestinal tract. The peak plasma level usually occurs within 1 to 3 hours after oral ingestion. The plasma half-life of clonazepam is 20 to 40 hours in adults and 15 to 33 hours in children. It is extensively metabolized in the liver to products which exhibit little, if any, pharmacological activity. These include 7-aminoclonazepam, 7-acetamidoclonazepam, 3-hydroxyclonazepam, 3-hydroxy-7-aminoclonazepam and 3-hydroxy-7-acetamidoclonazepam. The parent compound appears in the urine in amounts of less than 1 percent of the dose. About 80 percent of the drug in the plasma is bound to protein.[9,48]

Administration and Blood Levels The doses used in patients who benefitted from clonazepam have ranged from 0.1 to 0.2 mg/kg per day in children and 10 to 15 mg per day in adults. It is important to start with a relatively low dose, such as 0.01 to 0.03 mg/kg in children and 1.5 mg per day in adults, to avoid excessive sedation and unsteadiness at the onset of clonazepam therapy. The dose is then built up as tolerated until effective, or a maximum of 20 mg per day in adults. The blood levels in patients who benefitted from clonazepam have ranged from 20 to 70 nanograms/ml; levels over 80 nanograms/ml may be associated with excessive drowsiness. A dose of 10 mg per day in adults usually produces blood levels ranging from 25 to 35 ng/ml. The beneficial effects of clonazepam are often transient, lasting from 3 to 6 months to a year. Restarting after a period of "rest" for a few months may produce another period of improvement.[48]

Interactions Clonazepam administration has been noted to decrease phenytoin and primidone blood levels in some patients.[56]

Side Effects The high dose and blood level related side effects of clonazepam are sedation, fatigability and equilibrium disturbances. The initial sedative effect at the onset of therapy usually abates as tolerance to it develops. In some patients clonazepam, while controlling absence seizures or other minor seizure manifestations, seems to have precipitated generalized seizures.[48]

Skin rashes are extremely rare as are hematologic and hepatic complications in patients receiving clonazepam.

Diazepam

Chemical name: 7-chloro-1,3-dihydro-1-methyl-5-phenyl-2H-1,4-benzodiazepin-2-one

Proprietary names: Valium, Calmpose, Cercine, Freudal, Glorius, Lembrol, Seduxen, Tensopam and Valeo

Molecular weight: 284.76

Factor to convert concentration from ng/ml to nM is 3.5

Solubility in water: insoluble

Formulation and indications Diazepam is marketed as 2-, 5- and 10-mg tablets. Parenteral preparations are available as solutions in ampules containing 10 mg per 2 ml. It is an important drug in the treatment of status epilepticus, given intravenously.[10,43] It has also been used to treat myoclonic and akinetic seizures and infantile spasms.[9,35,63]

Mechanism of action Diazepam is effective against seizures induced either by electrical stimulation or pentylenetetrazol. It limits the spread of seizure discharges from a penicillin focus and raises the afterdischarge threshold in subcortical nuclei. The molecular mechanism of diazepam action is not well understood. An alteration of monoamine transmitter balance and turnover has been observed.[14,28]

Pharmacokinetic Parameters   Diazepam is well absorbed from the intestinal tract, the peak blood level occurring in 1 to 2 hours following oral ingestion. When given intravenously, it rapidly penetrates the blood-brain barrier resulting in high brain concentration within 2 to 10 minutes. Plasma half-life of diazepam is 10 to 25 hours.[8,19] Diazepam is relatively rapidly metabolized to N-desmethyl-diazepam, which also has antiepileptic properties and accumulates in the blood. The plasma half-life of desmethyl-diazepam ranges from 25 to 50 hours.[25] Further metabolites of diazepam include N-desmethyl-3-hydroxydiazepam, 2-hydroxydiazepam, oxazepam, 5-p-hydroxyphenyl-desmethyldiazepam and 5-p-hydroxyphenyl-diazepam.[15,28]

The majority of a dose can be recovered in the urine, where 3–5 percent of the dose appears as the parent compound, the rest as metabolites. About 95 percent of diazepam in the plasma is bound to proteins.[8]

Administration and Blood Levels   For the treatment of status epilepticus, diazepam is given intravenously. A dose of 10 mg usually stops the seizures. The effect may often last no longer than 20 to 30 minutes, then the dose is repeated. Caution is in order when giving diazepam intravenously, since too rapid administration may cause hypotension and respiratory depression. A rate of 2 mg per minute is adequate.[10,43]

In chronic treatment the doses used in children range from 1 to 5 mg per day; in adults from 15 to 40 mg per day given in divided doses. It is advisable to start with a low dose to alleviate sedation, which is common at the onset of therapy but later abates as tolerance develops. Blood levels of the parent compound in patients receiving 15 mg diazepam per day usually range from 150 to 250 ng/ml with concomitant levels of desmethyldiazepam ranging from 200 to 350 ng/ml. The sum total of the two compounds is probably the meaningful figure, as both are pharmacologically active. It is difficult to define effective and toxic blood level ranges in diazepam therapy because of the marked variations in tolerance among individuals as well as the development of tolerance in the same individual.

Interactions   Diazepam has caused elevation of phenytoin blood levels in some patients but had the opposite effect in others. In the majority of patients, however, no significant change of phenytoin blood level occurs after diazepam has been added to the medication regimen. Like phenytoin, it may alter the results of thyroid function tests but the patient usually remains euthyroid.[9,29,56]

Side Effects   Sedation, as mentioned above, is not an uncommon side effect of diazepam, and occurs in some patients with administration of a very low dose. Disturbance of equilibrium and coordination may also occur. Skin rashes, hematological complications and impairment of liver function are very rare.

Ethosuximide

Chemical name: 2-ethyl-2-methylsuccinimide

Proprietary names: Zarontin, Asamid, Emeside, Ethymal, Petinimid, Simatin among others

Molecular weight: 141.17

Factor   to convert concentration from μg/ml to μM is 7.08

Solubility in water: soluble

Formulation and Indications   Ethosuximide is marketed in the form of capsules (250 mg) and syrup (250 mg/5 ml). Parenteral preparations are not available. It is highly effective against absence seizures.

Mechanism of Action   Ethosuximide modifies synaptic transmission to low frequency electrical stimulation. It protects animals against pentylene-tetrazol-induced seizures, perhaps by affecting both the inhibitory and facilitatory neurons.[14,28,44]

Pharmacokinetic Parameters   Ethosuximide is readily absorbed, the peak blood level occurring within 1 to 4 hours of ingestion. Its biotransformation yields several oxidation products, excreted in the urine, which are all pharmacologically inactive. The plasma half-life is about 30 hours in children, and up to 60 hours in adults. Binding of ethosuximide to plasma proteins is practically nil.[15]

Administration and Blood Levels   Effective doses of ethosuximide range from 15 to 30 mg/kg per day, which is usually given in divided doses. Younger children tend to require higher doses in mg/kg than older children or adults. The dose can be built up relatively quickly if nausea and vomiting do not occur. The gastric irritation can be alleviated by taking the drug with a meal.

The maximal blood level from a given dose is reached within a week. Doses of 10 to 15 mg/kg usually render blood levels ranging from 20 to 50 μg/ml, 15 to 20 mg/kg results in 30 to 70 μg/ml, and 20 to 30 mg/kg results in

40 to over 100 μg/ml. Blood levels of less than 40 μg/ml are rarely effective. Levels up to 100 μg/ml are usually well tolerated. Levels well over 100 μg/ml may be associated with nausea, vomiting and sedation, although not always.[47,59]

Interactions   Interactions between ethosuximide and other drugs are extremely infrequent; rare cases of elevation of phenytoin blood levels have been reported.

Side Effects   Direct gastric irritation may occur initially with any dose. This is alleviated by taking the drug with a meal. High dose- and blood level-related side effects of ethosuximide are generally ill defined. Vomiting, sedation, headache, and ataxia are among them, but their occurrence shows marked variation among individuals.[59]

Skin rashes are infrequent but do occur, sometimes progressing to Stevens-Johnson syndrome. Depression of the hematopoietic system may occur, leukopenia being the most frequent manifestation, and pancytopenia the rarest. A few patients have developed lupus erythematosus while receiving ethosuximide.[54]

Ethosuximide in Pregnancy   Because ethosuximide is primarily used in children, experience in pregnancy is too limited to draw any conclusions.

Mephenytoin

Chemical name: 5-ethyl-3-methyl-5-phenylhydantoin

Proprietary names: Mesantoin, Epilan, Hidantin, Sedantoinal, Sacerno

Molecular weight: 218.5

Factor   to convert concentration from μg/ml to μM is 4.58

Solubility in water: insoluble

Formulation and Indications   Mephenytoin is marketed as 100 mg tablets. Parenteral preparations are not available. It is effective against generalized tonic-clonic and partial seizures. It is used sparingly because of relatively high incidence of toxic reactions.

Mechanism of action is probably similar to that of phenytoin.

Pharmacokinetic Parameters   Mephenytoin is well absorbed, the peak plasma level occurring 2 to 4 hours following ingestion. Time to reach steady state is 7

to 10 days. It is rapidly demethylated to 5-ethyl-5-phenylhydantoin (Nirvanol) which also has antiepileptic action. Plasma half-life of the parent compound is 1 to 2 days, that of ethyl-phenylhydantoin 2 to 3 days. The end-product of its biotransformation is 5-ethyl-5-parahydroxyphenyl-hydantoin. About 50 percent of the drug is bound to plasma protein.[51,66]

Administration and Blood Levels   Common clinical doses range between 300 to 500 mg daily in adults, 3 to 10 mg/kg in children. In the blood during steady state the concentration of ethyl-phenylhydantoin is 4 to 10 times higher than that of the parent compound. Although it is possible to measure the concentrations of the parent compound and the metabolite separately, it is technically easier to express the sum total of the two, which appears to be adequate for clinical purposes. The concentration of mephenytoin products with common effective doses range between 20 to 40 μg/ml; intoxication may occur with levels over 50 μg/ml.[66]

Interactions: none reported

Side Effects   Skin rashes are more common with mephenytoin than with other antiepileptic drugs. This is not surprising considering that it is biotransformed to ethyl-phenylhydantoin, identical to Nirvanol. Nirvanol, once used to treat Sydenham's chorea, has been long ago withdrawn from the market because of a high incidence of skin and other toxic reactions. Depression of hematopoietic functions are frequent, manifested by leukopenia, thrombocytopenia and aplastic anemia. On the other hand, gum hyperplasia and hirsutism, the common side effects of the structurally similar phenytoin, do not occur.[54,74]

Phenobarbital (Phenobarbitone)

Chemical name: 5-ethyl-5-phenyl-barbituric acid

Proprietary names: Alepsal, Fenemal, Gardenal, Laureal, Luminal, Phenemal among others

Molecular weight: 232.2

Factor   to convert concentration from μg/ml to μM is 4.3

Solubility in water: sodium salt freely soluble

Formulation and Indications   Phenobarbital is marketed as tablets of 15 to 100 mg. Liquid oral preparations are available, as well as ampules to be reconstituted for parenteral administration.

Phenobarbital is effective against generalized tonic-clonic and most partial seizures.

Mechanism of Action   Phenobarbital apparently exerts its antiepileptic action mainly by reducing the synaptic transmission of impulses non-selectively. This may result from alterations in the movement of ions across the cell membrane and changes in transmitter release.[14,28]

Pharmacokinetic Parameters   Phenobarbital is absorbed slowly from the intestinal tract, the peak blood level occurring within 5 to 15 hours. It undergoes biotransformation; recovery in urine from a dose is 20–40 percent for the parent compound and about the same amount for the hydroxy metabolites.[23] The excretion of the parent compound is pH dependent: alkalinization enhances the process and may be used in the treatment of overdose. The plasma half-life of phenobarbital is relatively long, about 2 to 5 days (average 3), and shorter in children than in adults. This may account in part for the need for higher mg/kg doses in children. Binding of phenobarbital to plasma protein is about 50 percent.[15,74]

Administration and Blood Levels   Average effective doses of phenobarbital in adults are 60 to 150 mg or 1 to 2 mg/kg per day; 3 to 5 mg/kg per day in children.[2,9,53,63] As a child becomes older the dosage requirement diminishes, and it equals that of the adult after reaching puberty. When starting with average maintenance doses, the onset of antiepileptic effect is relatively slow; therefore "loading" with double the dose for 2 to 3 days may be used if seizure frequency is high. The daily dose is often given in two to three installments, but may be given as a single dose, particularly later in the course of therapy when tolerance to the sedative effects has developed. Some sedation at the onset of treatment or following an increase of the dose often occurs, but usually abates within a few days or weeks. The drug is well absorbed from intramuscular injection sites if parenteral administration becomes necessary.

Due to long half-life and slow absorption, the phenobarbital blood levels are rather stable, showing small diurnal variations. The time to reach maximum blood levels with a given dose is usually 2 to 3 weeks. There is reasonably good correlation between the dose of phenobarbital and the blood level; 1 mg/kg producing approximately 10 μg/ml in blood. Upon increase of dosage, a relatively proportional rise of blood level occurs, and saturation kinetics resulting in a disproportionately high rise of blood level have not been observed. Effectiveness usually starts with levels near 20 μg/ml. Continued sedation may occur with levels over 40 μg/ml, though some patients develop tolerance to levels well above that.[2,31,74]

Interactions   Phenobarbital is an inducer of mixed function oxidases in the liver and thus may enhance the metabolism of other drugs taken concomitantly. A lowering effect on phenytoin blood levels has been observed in some patients, but this is rarely of clinical consequence. Shortening of the half-life of anticoagulants has been noted, but this is usually compensated by regulating the anticoagulant doses based on prothrombin time determinations.[29,56] The effect of phenobarbital upon steroid and calciferol metabolism is variable among patients and some require vitamin D supplements.[16]

Side Effects   One side effect related to high dose and blood levels is sedation, to which little if any further tolerance develops. The initial transient sedation mentioned as occurring with low blood levels at the onset of therapy is usually waited out. In some children, hyperactivity may occur, which may necessitate changing to another drug. School performances in some children may suffer after onset of phenobarbital therapy, particularly if relatively high doses are needed to control the seizures. Changing the medication may be in order in this situation. Diminished libido or delayed ejaculation is a complaint of some patients taking phenobarbital.

Skin rashes caused by phenobarbital are quite rare, as are hematologic complications, liver damage, and collagen diseases.[56,74]

Phenobarbital in Pregnancy   There is no experimental evidence that phenobarbital is teratogenic. There is no statistical evidence that phenobarbital causes more birth defects than the other anticonvulsants.

Phenytoin

Chemical name: 5,5-diphenylhydantoin

Proprietary names: Dilantin, Antisacer, Epanutin, Epelin, Hidantina, Labopal, Phenhydan, Ritmenal among others.

Molecular weight: 252.3

Factor   to convert concentration from μg/ml to μM is 3.96

Solubility in water: soluble at alkaline pH

Formulation and Indications   Phenytoin for oral ingestion is marketed as capsules (30 and 100 mg), tablets (50 mg), and a suspension. Parenteral preparations are available, usually as ampules to be reconstituted with a special diluent.

Phenytoin is effective against generalized tonic-clonic and most partial seizures.

Mechanism of Action   Understanding of the mechanism of action of phenytoin is still incomplete, but it appears that phenytoin prevents the spread of seizure discharges primarily by suppressing post-tetanic potentiation. Thus, it has a somewhat selective effect upon the hyperactive neurons and synapses in the path of the seizure discharges. This occurs at concentrations that do not significantly affect other normal synapses. The underlying molecular mechanism includes alterations of the transport of Na, K, and Ca ions across the cell membrane and related changes in the transmitter release.[14,28]

Pharmacokinetic Parameters   Phenytoin is absorbed at moderate speed from the intestinal tract, the peak blood levels occur between 4 to 8 hours after ingestion. The rate and completeness of absorption may vary, depending upon preparations, presence of chelating agents and individual disposition.

Phenytoin needs to undergo biotransformation prior to elimination, only 1–2 percent of the dose is excreted unchanged in the urine. Therefore it is vulnerable to any factor that can influence the rate or the total capacity of its metabolism. The determining factors are genetic make-up, status of liver function and presence of other drugs. Self-induction of phenytoin metabolism is minimal but other inducers may enhance it to a variable extent. The major metabolite is p-hydroxyphenylphenylhydantoin (HPPH) which is inactive and appears in the urine usually in an amount of 60–70 percent of the dose.[15,24,27] The latter measure is useful in evaluating absorption problems. Phenytoin metabolism is subject to saturation kinetics, resulting in accumulation and disproportionate rise of blood level if the saturation point is exceeded.[9,19,35]

Plasma half-life of phenytoin is dose-dependent, averaging around 20 hours, and it is shorter in children than in adults.[8,15]

In the plasma of normal adults about 90 percent of phenytoin is bound to plasma protein, less in younger children. In patients with chronic uremia or liver disease 80 percent or less may be bound.[45]

Administration and Blood Levels   Effective phenytoin doses range from 300 to 500 mg (4 to 6 mg/kg) per day in adults; 6 to 8 mg/kg in children.[2,9,40,53,72] The common starting dose of 300 mg daily in adults produces blood levels ranging from 5 to 15 μg/ml reached within 5 to 10 days from the onset of therapy.[2,74] If a more rapid response is desired, a loading dose of approximately 20 mg/kg or near 1000 mg may be given in the first 24 hours, followed by usual maintenance doses. This produces blood levels over 10 μg/ml by the second day. Side effects of a loading dose in the form of gastric irritation and dizziness occur, but are usually not intolerable.

If seizure control is inadequate with 300 mg, an increase to 400 mg daily usually produces a rise in blood levels to 10 to 20 μg/ml range. Because of saturation kinetics of phenytoin metabolism which may result in a sharp upswing of blood level with high doses, it is advisable to use small dosage increments, (25 or 50 mg), if blood level is already approaching 20 μg/ml. This can be done by adding a 100 mg capsule to be taken every other day or by using 50 mg tablets, which can easily be broken in half. The daily dose is usually given in 2 or 3 installments but can be taken all at once, if tolerated.[9]

In rare individuals the common phenytoin dose of 300 mg, instead of producing the usual blood level up to 15 μg/ml, may cause accumulation to over 30 μg/ml. This is caused by genetically determined low enzyme reserve and the patient may be termed as slow phenytoin metabolizer. In others, very low levels are seen with common doses, these patients are fast metabolizers.[27] Low levels of phenytoin relative to the dose are also common in chronic uremic patients. Here, the low protein binding allows rapid transport to liver and rapid elimination, which may be compounded by induction of liver enzymes by other uremic products.

Effective blood levels in the majority of adults start near 10 μg/ml.[2,9,31,39] In situations with decreased protein binding of phenytoin, such as in young children and in patients with chronic uremia or liver disease, lower values may be effective, presumably because more drug is free to penetrate into tissues.

Blood levels over 20 μg/ml may cause side effects; mild at first, in form of nystagmus and blurred vision. Disturbance of equilibrium and dizziness may also occur when the blood level approaches 30 μg/ml. This is usually the case when the blood level increases rapidly in a patient with no tolerance to phenytoin side effects. Levels over 40 μg/ml may also cause some sedation. The intensity of side effects with high blood levels varies among patients, in part because of tolerance; and it is not altogether rare to see patients free of symptoms with blood levels over 30 μg/ml. Nystagmus, although often seen with high blood levels, is not a reliable sign in children, in part perhaps, because children may not be able to sustain a fixed gaze upon test objects.[2,31]

The best route to administer phenytoin is orally, in capsule or tablet form. The oral suspension is difficult to manage, because it requires shaking before administration and even then the doses from the top of the bottle may be smaller than from the bottom of the bottle. A reasonably reliable way to administer phenytoin to small children is to crush a tablet in a spoon and mix with applesauce. If oral intake is impossible, phenytoin may be given intravenously or intramuscularly. Intravenous administration maintains the desired blood level, but needs to be carried out with precaution (see section on treatment of status epilepticus) and is cumbersome for prolonged therapy.[5,67,70] Intramuscular administration is the last resort because it is quite painful, may cause sterile abscesses, and the absorption from intramuscular deposits is erratic and delayed. Crystals of phenytoin at the site of intramuscular injection have been observed in experimental animals.[71]

Interactions   Because phenytoin elimination depends on its biotransformation, which is sensitive to a variety of agents, numerous drug-drug interactions have been observed.[29,56] Of clinical concern are those which may result in severe phenytoin intoxication from inhibition of its metabolism. Drugs that predictably cause marked elevation of phenytoin blood levels are disulfiram and sulthiame. Isoniazid causes predictably marked accumulation of phenytoin only in the very slow isoniazid inactivators. Other drugs potentially capable of inhibiting phenytoin metabolism are chloramphenicol, phenyramidol, bishydroxycoumarin, some sulfa-drugs and others listed in Table 2-2.

It is generally advisable to monitor phenytoin blood levels when a potentially interacting drug needs to be added. If a marked elevation of phenytoin blood level occurs, phenytoin dose should be reduced accordingly. The interaction usually becomes obvious within the first weeks or months of combined therapy; if no elevation occurs, there is little further concern. Small elevations of phenytoin level may be even beneficial in terms of seizure control.[29]

Phenobarbital as a hepatic enzyme inducer is theoretically expected to lower phenytoin blood levels. This has been observed in some patients, but in the majority no significant change occurs, and in others, phenobarbital causes some elevation of phenytoin blood level. This probably occurs because in addition to inducing, phenobarbital also competes with phenytoin for the enzyme, and the net effect then depends upon the balance between induction and inhibition. In general, there is little reason for concern about this effect in clinical settings.[29]

The other agents that may reduce phenytoin blood level, probably by

Table 2-2 / Drugs That May Cause Changes of Phenytoin Blood Level

Decrease	*Increase*	
	Predictable	*Sporadic*
Phenobarbital	Disulfiram	Methylphenidate
Carbamazepine	Sulthiame	Dicumarol
Tolbutamide	Isoniazid (slow inactivators)	Phenylbutazole
Ethanol		Sulfa drugs
DDT		Chloramphenicol
Diazepam		Phenothiazines
Clonazepam		Diazepam
		Phenobarbital

enhancing its metabolism, include carbamazepine, clonazepam and ethylalcohol. Calcium sulfate and antacids may lower phenytoin blood level by interfering with phenytoin absorption.

Phenytoin, in return, can lower the blood levels of anticoagulants, carbamazepine, digitoxin, DDT and endogenous and administered steroids, among others.[29,56]

Relevant Side Effects   High dose and blood level related side effects include blurred vision and nystagmus, dizziness, disturbance of equilibrium and, with very high levels, sedation. Permanent cerebellar damage from prolonged very high phenytoin concentrations is a possibility.

Gastric irritation is not common but may occur, particularly when attempt is made to administer the daily amount in one installment.

In up to 50 percent of patients, gum hyperplasia is to some extent caused by phenytoin. This is more likely to be severe when the drug is started at an early age in high doses and is generally alleviated by good oral hygiene. Sometimes surgical removal of excess tissue is necessary. The tissue proliferation rarely involves other facial structures resulting in leonine facies. Dupuytren's contracture is not infrequent in patients taking phenytoin. These manifestations are often accepted as an unfortunate, but unavoidable price for freedom from seizures, where phenytoin has thus far proven to be the best of all the tried agents for seizure control. Hirsutism is also relatively frequent and may be cosmetically disturbing, but clinically innocuous.[32,54]

Skin rashes occur in 1–5 percent of patients started on phenytoin. It is always advisable to stop the medication then, since some rashes have proceeded to exfoliative dermatitis or Stevens-Johnson syndrome. Later, phenytoin may be tried again and often the rash does not recur. Acute serum sickness-like picture occurs rarely and is treated with steroids.[54]

Lymphadenopathy including pseudolymphoma occurs in a small number of patients, but malignant lymphoma caused by phenytoin occurs rarely, if at all. Lupus erythematosus has been reported to occur in patients taking phenytoin. Depression of the hematopoietic system by phenytoin is very rare, with the exception of megaloblastic anemia. Liver damage is rare, occurring nearly always only as a part of generalized allergic reactions.[54]

Thyroid function tests (protein bound iodine, thyroxine levels) may be altered by phenytoin but the patients remain euthyroid and do not require thyroid therapy.[17]

Hyperglycemia has occurred in some patients from high phenytoin concentrations, presumably because phenytoin can block the release of insulin from the islet cells. Common clinically used doses and concentrations of phenytoin do not cause hyperglycemia or alter insulin release.[6]

Phenytoin can accelerate vitamin D metabolism[16] and lower serum folate levels[54] leading to a need for supplementation therapy, such as in patients with folate deficiency anemia or osteoporosis. Prophylactic administration of folic acid, 1 to 3 mg per day, is practiced by some physicians, others reserve its use for clearcut clinical indications. Prophylactic vitamin D supplementation is probably indicated only when the diet is deficient of the vitamin and/or exposure to sunlight is limited.[32,54]

Phenytoin in Pregnancy   Given in large doses to pregnant animals, phenytoin has caused cleft palate, cleft lip, and limb and organ anomalies in the offspring. Similar manifestations occur 2 to 3 times as often in babies born to mothers taking phenytoin alone or in combination with other antiepileptic drugs than in the general population.[20] (see Table 2-3). There is a growing concern about the teratogenecity of phenytoin in recent literature. The term "fetal hydantoin syndrome" has been coined as one in which manifestations, in addition to those mentioned above, include small head, large head, large eyes, wide-set eyes, and bushy hair among about 40 other signs and symptoms. The incidence of large, or wide-set eyes in control groups, however, is not known. Thus, the clinical significance of these inflated counts remains obscure. Of potential concern are observations that "phenytoin babies" may also show slow physical and mental development; further prospective studies are in order.[32]

There is little doubt that having epilepsy and needing to take phenytoin or other antiepileptic agents, increases the chances of having an abnormal baby from 2 percent in the general population to 6 percent as seen in the epileptic population. However, over 90 out of 100 babies born to epileptic mothers are normal. Since risks from seizures to mother and fetus outweigh the risk of teratogenecity, use of phenytoin in pregnancy will be continued until

Table 2-3 / Incidence of Birth Defects in General Population and in Epileptic Population Per 100 Births

	General population	Epileptics without medication	Epileptics on medication
Cleft lip and/or cleft palate	0.15%	*	1.8%
Heart defects	0.42%	1.0%	1.5%
Skeletal anomalies	*	*	1.0%
Other	*	*	2.2%
Totals	2.5%	4.2%	6.5%

*Data insufficient to calculate percentage
Adapted from Janz D: The teratogenic risk of antiepileptic drugs. Epilepsia 16: 159–169, 1975

new agents which are as effective, but totally free of teratogenic effects become available.[20]

Phenytoin quite rarely can cause vitamin K deficiency and a bleeding tendency in the neonate. This is treated with parenteral vitamin K, 5 mg three times a day. It is advisable to give the mother 5 mg of vitamin K prophylactically before delivery.[62]

Primidone

Chemical name: 2-desoxyphenobarbital

Proprietary names: Mysoline, Cyral, Dylon, Hexadonia, Liskantin, Midone, Mysedon

Molecular weight: 218.3

Factor   to convert concentration from μg/ml to μM is 4.58

Solubility in water: insoluble

Formulation and Indications   Primidone, a congener of phenobarbital, is marketed in tablet form, (250 mg and 50 mg) and as an oral suspension. Parenteral preparations are not available so far. It is effective against generalized tonic-clonic and most partial seizures.

Mechanism of Action   Evaluation of the mechanism of action of primidone is complicated by its conversion to phenobarbital and phenylethyl-malonamide (PEMA) after ingestion. The parent compound may have some effect and PEMA has been shown to possess antiepileptic properties. During chronic administration, the phenobarbital concentration in the body is higher than that of the parent compound or PEMA. It is thus likely that the major antiepileptic effect of primidone therapy comes from the derived phenobarbital and consists of modification of synaptic transmission.

Pharmacokinetic Parameters   Primidone is readily absorbed from the intestinal tract, peak plasma level of primidone occurs in 2 to 4 hours. Its plasma half-life is around 6 to 12 hours. As already mentioned, some of it is metabolized to phenyl-ethyl-malonamide (PEMA) and phenobarbital. The half-life of PEMA is 40 to 60 hours, and that of phenobarbital is over 72 hours. Elimination takes place via the kidneys. From a given dose, up to 50 percent is recovered in the urine as primidone, 5–15 percent as phenobarbital and its metabolites, and 10–25 percent as PEMA. The binding of primidone to plasma proteins is negligible.[8,15,74,75]

Administration and Blood Levels   The clinically common effective doses of primidone range from 750 to 1250 mg or 10 to 20 mg/kg daily. It is usually given in divided doses. Marked sedation and dizziness are reported by many patients if the therapy is initiated with the full dose. This can be avoided or alleviated by starting with half a tablet twice a day and building the dose up as tolerated. Tolerance usually develops to the initial side effects (which, are probably caused by primidone itself since the production of PEMA and phenobarbital is merely beginning during the first day or two). It has been suggested that primidone therapy is simply a more expensive form of phenobarbital therapy. This may hold true for some patients, but in others an improvement of seizure control has been seen when the medication was changed from phenobarbital to primidone.

During chronic administration of primidone, the phenobarbital blood level is usually 2 to 4 times higher than that of primidone. The blood level ratio of phenobarbital to primidone is usually lower when primidone is the only medication, and higher when another drug such as phenytoin is also used.[11] The PEMA blood level is equal to or somewhat higher than that of the parent compound. For the parent compound, the maximum level from a given dose is reached in a few days, in a week for PEMA, and after several weeks for phenobarbital. Due to the short half-life of primidone, its blood level shows marked diurnal variations depending on the time of ingestion of the last dose. A dose of 750 mg of primidone daily usually renders blood levels ranging from 15 to 30 μg/ml of phenobarbital and 5 to 10 μg/ml of primidone; 1000 mg daily may produce 20 to 40 μg/ml of phenobarbital and 7 to 15 μg/ml of primidone.[30] In evaluating blood level data during primidone therapy, the phenobarbital level is the most useful value. Its effective range starts near 20 μg/ml, and the concomitant primidone level is usually over 5 μg/ml. PEMA levels are rarely available, for technical reasons. Sedation and ataxia may be expected with phenobarbital levels of over 40 μg/ml and primidone levels of over 15 μg/ml, subject to the degree of individual tolerance. A very low phenobarbital level with a moderate or higher primidone level in a presumably chronically medicated patient, usually reflects irregular drug intake. In this case, the patient probably stops medication and then restarts a few days prior to the office visit.[19,31,74]

Interactions   Primidone therapy via the derived phenobarbital may induce the metabolism of a variety of drugs, though in clinical practice, no major effects of that nature are usually seen. Primidone metabolism may be enhanced by phenytoin[11] and inhibited by isoniazid.[65]

Side Effects   High dose and blood level-related side effects of primidone are mainly sedation, dizziness, ataxia, and blurred vision. Skin rashes occur but are not frequent, and depression of the hematopoietic system is rarely seen in the form of megaloblastic anemia, leukopenia, or thrombocytopenia. Lupus erythematosus has been also reported.[54]

Primidone in Pregnancy   There is no evidence that primidone is more likely than the other anticonvulsants to cause birth defects.

Valproate

Chemical names: di-N-propylacetate; 2-propylpentanoate

Proprietary names: Depakene, Convulex, Epilim, Ergenyl, Logical, Atemperator

Molecular weight: free acid: 144; sodium salt: 166

Factor   to convert concentration from μg/ml to μM is 6.4

Solubility in water: soluble

Formulation and Indications   Valproic acid and its sodium salt are among the newest effective antiepileptic agents. Valproate is marketed as foil-packed tablets (because of the hygroscopic nature of the material), capsules, and syrup. Currently, only oral preparations are available. It is quite effective against absence seizures and other spike-and-wave epilepsies and also has some beneficial effect against generalized tonic-clonic and partial complex seizures.[49]

Mechanism of Action   The mechanism of action of valproate may be in part related to its ability to elevate gamma-amino-butyric acid concentrations in the brain by influencing the activity of the GABA-transaminase.[49,60] Other mechanisms may also be involved, including an active metabolite with a long plasma half-life.

Pharmacokinetic Parameters   Valproate is rapidly absorbed from the intestinal tract. Peak plasma levels usually occur between 1 to 4 hours, averaging 2 hours, following ingestion. Its plasma half-life is short, 6 to 12 hours, making it necessary to divide the daily dose into at least three installments. The known metabolites that are found in the urine include 2-n-propyl-5-hydroxy-pentanoic acid and 2-n-propylglutaric acid.[49,58] An active, circulating, as yet unidentified metabolite which is eliminated slowly is also thought to exist. Elimination takes place mostly via the kidney. About 90 percent of valproate in the blood is bound to plasma proteins. It passes the placenta and is found in the breast milk of nursing mothers. [49,60]

Administration and Blood Levels   Doses of valproate that have been effective in patients with absence and other spike-and-wave epilepsies have ranged from 15 to 50 mg/kg, average 25 mg/kg per day, taken in three installments. It is advisable to start with a low dose, approximately 10 mg/kg, though, because of frequently occurring initial gastric irritation. The dose may then be built up as tolerated by adding a capsule or a teaspoonful, perhaps, every 3 to 7 days until it appears that maximum benefit has been achieved. If severe nausea or vomiting occurs, the dose should be reduced until symptoms disappear, then a cautious increase at a slower rate may be attempted again. The most practical division of the daily dose consists of giving the first installment in the early morning and the last before bedtime, spacing the middle installment in between. Many of the patients in whom valproate is started are those who are already taking ethosuximide, but continue having absence seizures. If valproate stops their seizures, it is reasonable to attempt to withdraw ethosuximide. This can be done successfully in some patients, but others seem to do better with combination therapy, though the amount of ethosuximide can then be reduced.[49,60]

Generalized tonic-clonic or partial complex seizures, if they respond to valproate, require about the same dosages as absence seizures. In this setting, valproate is usually used as an add-on drug to barbiturates, hydantoins, or carbamazepine, which have been only partly effective, even at high doses. Addition of valproate may considerably diminish the number of seizures in these patients, and allow them to reduce the intake of other medications. This is of practical importance in patients whose barbiturate dosage had to be kept high, with concomitant sedation.[49,60]

Because of rapid absorption, short plasma half-life, and the use of divided doses, the valproate blood level shows greater diurnal variations than most other antiepileptic drugs. Yet, if the blood sample is always taken at the same time of day, preferably before the morning dose from in-patients, useful information can be gained from valproate blood levels. Regarding the dose-blood level relationship, a dose of 20 mg/kg generally produces blood levels between 30 to 60 μg/ml; 30 mg/kg produces 40 to 80 μg/ml, and 50 mg/kg produces 50 to 120 μg/ml. Regarding effectiveness, levels less than 40 μg/ml are rarely beneficial and levels near 100 μg/ml are usually tolerated well. Potentially toxic levels are probably well over 100 μg/ml.

Interactions   Valproate diminishes phenobarbital elimination, possibly by interfering with its excretion. Thus, in patients who are taking phenobarbital or a phenobarbital producing drug such as primidone, mephobarbital, or eterobarbital, the phenobarbital blood level will rise after valproate has been started. Monitoring the phenobarbital blood level and adjusting the barbiturate dosage as necessary is mandatory to avoid extreme sedation. Occasionally, alteration of phenytoin blood levels may also occur after addition of valproate, but this is less predictable and rarely requires a change in phenytoin dosage.[49,60]

Relevant Side Effects   The most common side effects, as already alluded to, are gastric discomfort, nausea, and vomiting. There are two types of nausea and vomiting caused by valproate. The first occurs soon after the ingestion of the drug, probably from direct gastric irritation. This may be experienced by up to one third of the patients started on valproate, but tolerance develops within a few days. The second type of nausea and vomiting occurs 1 to 3 hours following ingestion, coinciding apparently with the peak blood level, and is probably of central origin. This is more rare and sometimes abates gradually, but may persist and necessitate discontinuation of the drug.

Sedation attributable to valproate alone, in contradistinction to sedation caused by increasing phenobarbital concentration on combination therapies, occurs quite rarely. It may or may not abate with time.

Other rarely observed events are transient loss of hair and bleeding tendency. The latter is thought to result from altered platelet function; therefore periodical platelet counts are advisable. Occasionally, excessive weight gain occurs in some patients; this could be of concern in cosmetic but hardly in medical terms.[49,60]

Of serious concern, however, is the very rarely occurring impairment of liver functions which has resulted in a few fatalities. It is usually not a rapid hypersensitivity reaction, but appears to be dose-related and is heralded by gradual elevations of SGOT and SGPT. The liver function should be monitored in the early phase and during dosage regulations of valproate therapy, and the dosage should be reduced or discontinued when SGOT and SGPT become markedly elevated. It is probable that significant liver function impairment by valproate occurs mostly in those patients who are taking other drugs in large amounts and whose liver is already under a heavy load. Thus, in some patients on combination therapy, SGOT and SGPT became moderately elevated after a valproate dose increase, but returned to normal after valproate dose reduction. If, then, the dose of other drugs was reduced, the valproate dose could be increased without recurrence of SGOT and SGPT elevation. This is of practical importance in patients whose seizure control was incomplete with the other medication and who seemed to benefit considerably from the addition of valproate.

Valproate in Pregnancy   Valproate given experimentally in large amounts to pregnant animals has caused fetal abnormalities. It is not yet known whether

Table 2-4 / Additional Antiepileptic Drugs

	Effective against	Common daily doses (mg)	T/2	Blood levels[1] (μg/ml)
Mephobarbital	GTC[2]	200–500	short	low
AM[3]			3–5 days	10–30 μg/ml
Metharbital	GTC[2]	300		
Methsuximide	W[4]	900	11–12 hrs	less than 1 μg/ml
AM[3]			24–48 hrs	20–50 μg/ml
Nitrazepam	A[5]	10–25	10–20 hrs	
Phenacetamide	GTC[2]	1500		
Phensuximide	W[4]	1000	4–8 hrs	4–8 μg/ml
AM[3]			short	1–2 μg/ml
Sulthiame	GTC[2]	400–800	8 hrs	4–8 μg/ml

[1] Blood levels observed with common clinical doses.
[2] Generalized tonic-clonic seizures
[3] Active metabolites
[4] Wide spectrum
[5] Absence

clinical doses would do the same in human practice. Thus, its use during pregnancy remains a matter of judgement at the present time.

For additional antiepileptic drugs, see Table 2-4.

TREATMENT OF EPILEPSIES

Basic Considerations

Drugs that "cure" epilepsy once and for all do not exist, yet. The currently used antiepileptic agents merely prevent the seizures from occurring and that, only when they are present at the site of action in active form. Their effects are generally related to their concentration. The antiepileptic effects are usually achieved with concentrations that are lower than those causing intoxication. The concentration of drugs that are necessary to suppress or prevent the seizures vary among individual patients considerably, probably because of variations in the intensity of the seizure process. Thus one of the important tasks for the successful management of seizures is to match the severity of the seizure process with effective concentrations of appropriate drugs.

The selection of the drug is based on the type of seizures exhibited. Generalized tonic-clonic and partial seizures respond best to hydantoins, barbiturates and carbamazepine. Absence seizures respond best to succinimides, valproate and oxazolidinediones. Myoclonic and other early childhood seizures respond best to benzodiazepines and steroids. Selection of a drug among those effective against a seizure type is based upon the relative toxicity and the nature of the side effects of the drug. Thus, phenytoin may be preferred over barbiturates because its cosmetic side effects may be considered less disturbing than the sedation from barbiturates.

It is always wise to start therapy with one drug rather than with combinations.[55] This is preferable for following reasons: (1) A single drug may be all the patient needs. (2) If a skin rash, or other idiosyncratic complications occur, there is no question as to which drug is causing it. (3) There will be other drugs to choose from, if the first one is ineffective.

If the response to the first drug is considered unsatisfactory despite adequate blood concentrations, a second drug has to be added. The decision as to whether or not to continue the first drug, depends upon the effectiveness of the second drug and the degree of benefit that was observed from the first drug alone. In patients with a severe seizure process, a combination is needed. Administration of more than three drugs at a time is rarely practical. Discontinuation of antiepileptic drugs should be gradual. Withdrawal seizures are most likely to occur following abrupt cessation of barbiturates.

Use of Blood Levels

The rationale for use of blood levels was discussed in a previous section and is reviewed here. Correlations of clinical and laboratory data indicate that with most major antiepileptic drugs, blood levels that are effective in suppressing or controlling seizures in the majority of patients, are above a certain range.[2,8,26,30,39,50] These blood level ranges can be used as general guidelines at the initiation of therapy, followed by adjustments in individual patients as needed, according to the severity of the seizure process. Similarly, ranges of blood levels can be defined in which the majority of patients is expected to start showing evidence of intoxication. The development of tolerance becomes a factor here, and a level that initially was associated with intoxication may not exert that effect later. However, the concepts of "effective" and "toxic" blood level ranges are helpful in making clinical decisions in following the progress of individual patients during the course of therapy. There is also a correlation between the dose and blood level: low doses generally produce low levels, high doses produce high levels. However, because of individual variations in the pharmacokinetic parameters, the blood levels produced by the same dose may vary considerably among individuals. This makes it necessary to ascertain what level a patient will have with an individual dose. Furthermore, the dose and blood level relationship is not always linear; with an increase of the dose, self-induction may reduce the expected rise in the blood level; whereas, reaching saturation kinetics may cause a sharp upswing of the blood level. The saturation point of biotransformation is crucial with drugs that are not eliminated in an unchanged form, such as phenytoin; and the height of the saturation varies among individuals. Allowing for all these factors, however, it is possible to define ranges of blood levels that are expected to occur with a given dose in the majority of patients (Table 2-5). The concept of expected level ranges from a dose allows us to recognize and evaluate problems associated with levels that are too low or too high relative to the dose. These problems include possible noncompliance, drug interactions and unusual rates of drug absorption and elimination.

When to Order Blood Level Determinations   The established antiepileptic drugs have relatively long plasma half-lives, thus reaching the steady state takes time (approximately 5 times the half-life). See Table 2-5. Ordering blood levels too early may indicate whether a low or high range steady state is forthcoming, but does not indicate the maximum level to be achieved.

Generally, ordering blood levels can be useful in the following instances:

(1) After the onset of therapy, to ascertain what level the patient will get with a given dose; and the individual's effective level, if therapy is effective.

(2) After a change of dosage.

(3) After addition of new drugs, either antiepileptic or other, particularly if the addition is a potentially interacting drug.

(4) Inadequate seizure control.

(5) In the presence of signs and symptoms of intoxication, particularly if several drugs are taken.

(6) Periodically during the course of therapy to reinforce compliance. The patient now knows that he can be checked by the blood test.

Table 2-5 / Dose and Blood Level Relations and Times to Reach Steady State

Drug	Average dose (mg/day)	Expected level range (μg/ml)	Time to reach steady state (days)
Phenytoin	300	5–20	5–10
Phenobarbital	120	10–30	14–21
Primidone	750	5–15	3–5
Carbamazepine	1,200	4–12	4–6
Ethosuximide	750	20–70	4–8
Trimethadione	900	300–800 (as DMO)	30–60
Diazepam	15	0.1–0.3	4–6
Clonazepam	4	0.015–0.050	4–6
Valproate	1,000	30–90	2–3

What Blood Levels to Order   With phenytoin, phenobarbital, ethosuximide and valproate, the parent compound is the active principle. Active metabolites, which are more important than the rapidly metabolized parent compound, are produced by trimethadione, mephenytoin, mephobarbital and methsuximide. Primidone produces two active metabolites: phenylethylmalonamide and phenobarbital.

When to Draw Blood   Samples should be obtained about the same time of day if serial follow-up is planned, since some diurnal variations may occur. An early morning sample drawn before the first dose will represent the lowest point of the curve.

Plasma versus Serum   There is no difference in the drug concentration between serum and plasma. From the laboratory point of view, plasma is easier to separate than serum. Severe hemolysis tends to reduce the values for most drugs, therefore it is advisable to separate plasma or serum before storage.

How to Store the Samples   Freezing is not necessary except when long storage (weeks or months) is planned. Standing overnight, or for several days at room temperature does not alter the drug concentration values. For short term storage, a 4° temperature is adequate. Refrigeration is not necessary when mailing.

Units in Laboratory Reports   Most values in the literature have been given in μg/ml. Reporting in mg/liter gives the same numerical values as μg/ml. If reporting in mg per 100 ml, the number is 10 times smaller than μg/ml. If the report is in μM, the number is 4–6 times that of μg/ml. The conversion factor μg/ml to μM is derived by dividing *one* (1) by the molecular weight of the drug and multiplying by one thousand.

Clinical Considerations

A thorough diagnostic evaluation is necessary in all patients presenting with a recent onset of seizures. The major concerns are the following:

(1) Are the episodes really seizures that would respond to treatment with antiepileptic drugs (rather than syncope, hysterical manifestations, etc.)

(2) Is there a brain lesion present that requires specific treatment, such as brain tumor or abscess.

(3) Are the seizures caused by some toxic mechanism (phenothiazines, in rare susceptible individuals) or metabolic mechanisms (pyridoxine deficiency).

Recognition of the episodes as real seizures is usually not difficult, if accurate description is available and characteristic electroencephalographic findings are present. Discovery of a brain tumor may escape the initial work-up if the tumor is small. Therefore, patients with seizures starting in adulthood should have periodic reevaluation, particularly if the seizures are focal in nature and increase in frequency despite adequate antiepileptic drug therapy. The possibility of toxic or metabolic mechanisms being involved is usually clarified by the initial work-up.[9,63]

When to Start Therapy

Once the decision is made based on the initial evaluation that the seizures are of the kind that respond to antiepileptic drugs, there is a rational base for starting the therapy.[9] Whether or not to treat a patient who has had a single seizure, has been debated, mainly because the drugs have side effects and expose the patient to some risk. It appears practical, however, to treat an adult patient after his first generalized tonic-clonic seizure, simply because his next one may be his last one, if it occurs while swimming or driving a car, for instance. Some partial and absence seizures are less urgent because of their mild nature, and treatment is often delayed because the patient comes to the physician only when the episodes become disturbingly frequent. The latter course in itself indicates that waiting does not solve the problem and early treatment in these types of disorders seems also to be indicated. Thus, it appears reasonable that once the diagnosis of epilepsy is made, the therapy should be started.

Prophylactic treatment of children who have had febrile seizures has been reported to reduce the chances of development of non-febrile seizure disorders in later life.[37,73]

Precautions

Most antiepileptic drugs may occasionally cause depression of hematopoietic system functions. Leukopenia, neutropenia, thrombocytopenia as well as megaloblastic anemia have been reported to occur in some patients. What makes these patients vulnerable, is not known. This complication in susceptible individuals tends to become manifest within the first six months from the onset of therapy, sometimes later. In some patients the initial drop in the white cell count may revert spontaneously, in others, lowering of the dose may be necessary. If the blood counts continue to drop (white count less than 3,000; polymorphonuclear cells less than 1,800 and platelets less than 100,000), the drug should be discontinued.

Skin rashes have occurred with most of the currently used antiepileptic drugs in some patients. When a patient is started on a previously untried drug, he should be told that a skin rash may occur and that he should contact the physician immediately, if this happens. If not instructed to do so, the patient may assume that it is an insignificant, expected nuisance. It is safest to stop the medication whenever a rash occurs because sometimes (though very rarely) a simple morbilliform rash may develop further into an exfoliative dermatitis. If the drug is stopped, the rash always subsides. After a month or two, the same drug may be tried again, if it seemed highly effective during the first trial. The rash may then not occur, but if it does, the drug should be stopped and not used again. Administration of antihistaminics and calamine lotion is appropriate during the rash.

Impairment of liver function is another infrequent but potentially dangerous manifestation occurring with antiepileptic drugs. A rise in serum SGOT and SGPT usually precedes the rise of bilirubin and clinical jaundice. The incidence of this complication is low but warrants periodic monitoring of liver function tests.[54]

Treatment of Tonic-Clonic Seizures (Primary or Secondary Grand Mal)

The aim in treating generalized tonic-clonic seizures is to stop them or reduce their occurrence to a minimum. Each such seizure may have severe consequences if it takes place, for instance, while swimming, climbing steep stairs or operating a motor vehicle.

For the treatment of either primary or partial secondary generalized tonic-clonic seizures, the drugs phenytoin, phenobarbital, primidone and carbamazepine are effective. Phenytoin is the drug of choice, because it does not cause sedation in effective doses and seldom causes serious complications. In many adult patients, 300 to 400 mg daily is a satisfactory dose, but in very rare occasions, as little as 100 mg or as much as 600 mg may be needed. This variation occurs, firstly, because of variations in the efficacy of phenytoin metabolism among individuals, as pointed out in the section "Phenytoin". Thus the same dose may maintain low, average or high concentrations depending upon the individual's disposition. Secondly, the severity of the seizure process varies among individuals, requiring different concentrations for its control.

Generally, the aim of treatment is to achieve a phenytoin blood level of 10 μg/ml or slightly higher. This is practical because it appears that the severity of the seizure process in many patients is then matched with an effective drug concentration.[2,31] This phenytoin concentration range may be more than what is needed for patients with a low intensity seizure process but it is always well tolerated and thus not harmful. For patients with a severe seizure process, the phenytoin dose needs to be increased to reach blood levels near 20 μg/ml or slightly higher.[39] Increasing the phenytoin dose in patients with blood level approaching 20 μg/ml is best done in 25 or 50 mg installments to avoid passing the saturation point of the drug's metabolism and causing a marked upswing of the blood level which is disproportionate to the dose.[9]

If seizure control remains inadequate with phenytoin levels near 25 μg/ml, the dose should be reduced and a second drug added. The second drug could be phenobarbital (45 to 120 mg daily), or primidone (750 mg daily), building up the dose slowly. The barbiturate dose may be built up further, if needed, to yield phenobarbital blood levels of over 20 μg/ml, whether from phenobarbital itself or derived from primidone. Reaching phenobarbital levels of over 40 μg/ml often slows the patient down and may not significantly improve the seizure control. Primidone blood level should range from 5 to 15 μg/ml in the effective nontoxic range. Addition of carbamazepine in doses of 600 to 1200 mg daily has benefited some hard-to-control patients with generalized tonic-clonic seizures.

In other hard-to-control patients who did not respond to the above regimens, mephenytoin in doses of 300 to 500 mg daily has been helpful;[66] valproate in doses of 1000 to 2000 mg daily may be tried.[49] Adding diazepam in doses of 7.5 to 15 mg daily may benefit those patients whose seizures are precipitated by tension and anxiety. If seizures tend to occur around menstrual periods, taking an extra pill of regular medication at that time may be helpful, as well as taking acetazolamide 250 to 500 mg daily for a week.

Some physicians, particularly in pediatric practice, prefer phenobarbital as the first choice for the treatment of generalized tonic-clonic seizures. This would eliminate the cosmetic side effects of phenytoin, namely gum hyperplasia and hirsutism. If used alone, the phenobarbital dose is 5 to 10 mg/kg in younger children, and 2 to 5 mg/kg in older children and adults. Sedation is the limiting factor in dosing. Hyperkinetic symptoms occur in some children and may necessitate change of medication, if persistent and severe.

Primidone, if used alone, is given in doses of 750 to 1500 mg daily. As with phenobarbital, the limiting factor in dosing is sedation.

Carbamazepine, if used alone, is given in doses of 800 to 1600 mg daily.

Treatment of Partial Complex (Temporal Lobe) Seizures

In the treatment of partial complex seizures, one has three choices for the primary drug: carbamazepine, phenytoin, and primidone. Phenytoin and primidone, often in combination, have been the mainstay in the treatment of this form of seizure.[63] However, carbamazepine, a relative newcomer, appears to be at least as effective as phenytoin or primidone and it has the advantage of causing less sedation than primidone in patients requiring high doses.[9,61]

If using phenytoin or primidone, one should follow the same principles as outlined under treatment of generalized tonic-clonic seizures.

If carbamazepine is used as a single drug, the effective dose may range from 800 to 1400 mg daily, taken best in three or four installments due to its relatively short plasma half-life. The aim is to achieve blood levels of over 5

μg/ml or even higher in patients with a severe seizure process. Blood levels of over 12 μg/ml are likely to cause blurred vision, disturbance of equilibrium, sedation, and headaches. Depression of bone marrow and liver damage have also been of concern with carbamazepine, perhaps more so than with hydantoins and barbiturates. Therefore, it is advisable to monitor blood counts and liver function tests, initially every month and after increasing the dose, later every three to six months, if the results are found stable. In patients not responding satisfactorily to the above three drugs, valproate may be added in doses of 1000 to 2000 mg daily. Other drugs occasionally helpful in hard-to-control patients with partial complex seizures include methsuximide (900 mg daily),[64] phenacetamide (750 mg daily; watch for liver damage), acetazolamide if seizure frequency is high during menstrual periods, benzodiazepines, and phensuximide (1000 mg daily).[52]

In general, achieving complete control of partial complex seizures is often not an easy task and one may have to compromise between maximum reduction of seizure frequency and minimum side effects from medications. Fortunately, the milder forms of episodes in this disorder and those which are ameliorated by treatment are often not too disruptive. The patient may learn to live with them and be able to function in his occupation. He could be the judge of whether the disturbance caused by his seizures is greater or smaller than the side effects of high doses of medication, and the compromise treatment schedule could be adjusted accordingly.

Treatment of Absence (Petit Mal) Seizures

For the treatment of absence seizures, the first choice drug in the past decade has been ethosuximide. The effective doses have ranged from 750 to 1500 mg daily in adults and 10 to 20 mg/kg in children. The incidence of absence seizures is highest in the age group of 4 to 20 years. Young children often have difficulties with swallowing the capsule; for them the drug is given in the form of a syrup containing 50 mg per 1 ml. The maximum blood level from a given dose is reached within 7 to 10 days, and levels of over 40 μg/ml and up to 100 μg/ml are usually seen in patients with good clinical response.[47,59] Side effects in the form of nausea and vomiting occur at times and are usually alleviated by taking the drug with a meal or by reduction of dosage. Sedation is rare and may occur with high doses. Defining toxic blood level of ethosuximide is difficult because of the variability of side effects; it probably would be over 100 μg/ml.[31,47,59] Side effects of concern are skin rashes and depression of the hematopoietic system. Leukopenia is not infrequent and aplastic anemias have been reported. Therefore, blood counts should be monitored monthly for the first year of therapy, and later every three months.

A certain percentage (about 50 percent) of children with petit mal have or may start having generalized tonic-clonic seizures as well, particularly if the onset of absence seizures occurs around 10 years of age. Therefore, phenobarbital or phenytoin are often used concomitantly with ethosuximide. The phenobarbital dose in younger children is then 5 to 10 mg/kg, and 2 to 5 mg/kg in older children. Phenytoin is used in dosages of 5 to 10 mg/kg.[9,63]

Probably as effective as ethosuximide in the treatment of absence seizures is the newcomer valproate.[49,60] It may be used by itself or added to ethosuximide in those patients whose seizure control remains incomplete with ethosuximide alone. The effective doses of valproate range from 20 to 50 mg/kg, given as syrup or capsules in three divided doses. The maximum blood level with a dose is reached within a week, with effective blood level ranging from 50 to 120 μg/ml. Valproate often causes gastric irritation at the onset of therapy, which can be alleviated by taking it with meals or by temporarily reducing the dosage.[49,60]

If used together with phenobarbital, valproate causes phenobarbital accumulation. Therefore, phenobarbital blood levels need to be monitored and the dosage adjusted if excessive accumulation occurs. Serious side effects with valproate are less common than with most other antiepileptic drugs. Skin rashes and depression of the hematopoietic system are exceedingly rare, while a bleeding tendency with impaired platelet function has been reported on rare occasions. Impairment of liver function may occur. The liver damage seems to occur mostly when other drugs are also taken in large amounts and it is indicated by a rise of SGOT and SGPT values in liver function tests. These should be monitored monthly at the onset of therapy; and later, less often.

Trimethadione preceded ethosuximide as the first specific anti-absence agent. Although quite effective in terms of seizure control, it is used sparingly at the present time because of a relatively high incidence of toxic reactions, including kidney, liver, and hematopoietic damage. It serves as a substitute if ethosuximide or valproate can not be taken. The effective doses of trimethadione range from 900 to 1500 mg per day in adults and 20 to 40 mg/kg in children. Trimethadione (TMO) is rapidly metabolized to dimethadione (DMO), which is the pharmacologically active compound of importance in trimethadione therapy. The maximum blood level of DMO with a given dose of TMO is reached within a month. The DMO blood level in patients with a satisfactory clinical response ranges from 600 to 1000 μg/ml. The toxic levels of DMO are probably well over 1000 μg/ml. The TMO blood levels are usually about 10 times less than the concomitant DMO levels. TMO levels are higher than DMO levels only in the first few days following the onset of therapy.[1,3]

If the response to ethosuximide, valproate, or trimethadione has been unsatisfactory, then acetazolamide, benzodiazepines, amphetamine, or a ketogenic diet may be tried.

In the majority of patients who started having absence seizures at an early age, the episodes tend to subside by the time they reach 20 years of age. The anti-absence medications can then be stopped by gradually reducing the dose over several months if no seizures have occurred in 2 years.

Treatment of Myoclonic Seizures

The various forms of myoclonic seizures (minor motor, infantile spasms, and akinetic, of the old nomenclature) have been and still are the most difficult to treat.

Steroid therapy has been successful to some extent in a fair number of patients with infantile spasms. ACTH may be given 20 to 40 units intramuscularly every day for 4 to 6 weeks. An alternative treatment is 2 mg/kg of prednisone continued for 1 to 2 months if improvement seems to take place with this regimen. Steroids should be tapered gradually at the end of the course.[9,33,63]

Ethosuximide and trimethadione usually have little if any effect in patients with myoclonic seizures. However, benzodiazepines have been helpful, at least temporarily.[33] Diazepam may be used in doses of 2 to 30 mg per day, depending upon individual response and tolerance. The limiting side effect in diazepam dosing is usually sedation. Clonazepam may also produce periods of improvement in patients with myoclonic seizures, which often last longer than those caused by diazepam.[48] Clonazepam is started at doses of 0.01 to 0.03 mg/kg and gradually built up to 0.2 mg/kg. The slow start is necessary to minimize the sedative side effects. In some patients, clonazepam has reduced the myoclonic seizures, but has caused other major generalized seizure manifestations to occur. Clonazepam blood levels have ranged from 20 to 60 nanograms/ml in patients who benefit from this drug. Damage to liver, kidney and hematopoietic systems is exceedingly rare with benzodiazepines, as are skin rashes.[48]

Valproate has also shown promise as an agent to be tried in patients with myoclonic seizures. Administration and dosing for these seizure types are the same as in treatment of absence seizures.

Treatment of Status Epilepticus

Status epilepticus is a condition in which seizures follow one another in close intervals, and the patient does not regain a usual state of awareness in between these seizures. It may occur with any seizure type: generalized tonic-clonic, partial complex, or absence. Status epilepticus of the generalized tonic-clonic type is a medical emergency because permanent brain damage may occur, presumably from anoxia and depletion of cerebral energy resources. Status epilepticus of the generalized tonic-clonic type may be caused by head trauma, brain abscess or other infection, or a sudden discontinuance of antiepileptic drugs, particularly in the case of the barbiturates. Metabolic causes such as hypoglycemia are to be distinguished in patients with repetitive seizures and treated accordingly.[46]

In the treatment of status epilepticus, there are two primary concerns: to maintain and secure adequate pulmonary ventilation and to stop the seizures as soon as possible. For the latter reason, the selected drugs are given intravenously. Shortacting barbiturates, such as amobarbital in a narcotizing dose of 1000 mg usually stop the seizures but also cause deep stupor. This is objectionable if the neurological signs need to be followed, as in patients with a head trauma or brain abscess. The seizures can be stopped without severe depression of nervous system functions by the use of diazepam or phenytoin. A satisfactory plan is to give 10 mg of diazepam intravenously over 3 to 5 minutes, which stops the seizures by the time the injection is completed.[9,10,43,63] If the effect of diazepam is short-lived, as it often is, it should be repeated and followed with an infusion of phenytoin in a loading dose of 25 mg/kg in children; 20 mg/kg or 750 to 1500 mg in adults.[5,67,70] This phenytoin dose usually produces blood levels of over 10 μg/ml which will remain in the effective range until the next day, when regular maintenance doses should be continued. Phenytoin should be infused slowly, no more than 50 mg per minute, while monitoring respiration, blood pressure, and EKG. Too rapid an administration of phenytoin may cause respiratory and cardiac arrest, particularly in elderly patients.[67] Phenytoin in the above large dosage is often effective by itself in stopping the seizures, but its administration takes at least 20 minutes: therefore it is practical to stop the seizures first with diazepam. Some physicians prefer phenobarbital as the maintenance therapy, particularly in pediatric practice. In this case, after the seizures have been stopped with diazepam, phenobarbital is given intramuscularly in doses of 5 to 10 mg/kg depending on the patient's age.

If the above regimens are ineffective in stopping status epilepticus of generalized tonic-clonic seizures, then ether or shortacting barbiturate anesthesia may have to be used. Some success in stopping status epilepticus that failed to respond to diazepam, amobarbital and phenytoin has been achieved with the use of chlormethiazole. This drug has the thiazole nucleus of thiamine, possesses sedative and anticonvulsant properties and is being used in the treatment of eclampsia and alcohol withdrawal. It has a very short half-life, 1 to 3 hours. When used for the treatment of status epilepticus, it may be given intravenously as 0.8% solution at a rate of 0.3 to 0.7 g per hour for a total dose of 3 to 5 g per day. Side effects include drowsiness, depression of respiration, increased bronchial secretions and stuffiness of the nose.

Usually, status epilepticus of absence and partial seizures also responds to intravenously given diazepam. However, in case of partial seizures, phenytoin or phenobarbital may have to be used as well.

Epilepsy and Pregnancy

In recent years, there has been increasing concern among physicians and to some extent among patients about the teratogenicity of antiepileptic drugs.

Statistical surveys indicate that babies born to mothers who have epilepsy have a greater chance of having birth defects than babies born to non-epileptic mothers. These defects include cleft lip, cleft palate, cardiac anomalies, intestinal atresias, and limb abnormalities.[20] It is not entirely clear to what extent the genetic background, the seizures and the antiepileptic medication contribute to these manifestations but each may have its share. The incidence of birth defects in the general population is about 2.5 percent. This figure is increased to 4.2 percent in the offspring of mothers who have epilepsy but do not take antiepileptic medication. The mechanical events and anoxia during a seizure may play a role here. The incidence of birth defects in the offspring of mothers who take antiepileptic drugs increases to 6.5 percent. This increase may then possibly, but not conclusively, be ascribed to the medication. Most of these mothers had been on combinations of several drugs, therefore, it is difficult to establish from the clinical data whether one drug could be distinctly more teratogenic than another. By what mechanism antiepileptic drugs might cause birth defects is not clear. One of the postulated mechanisms is the reduction of folate level, since antifolates such as methatrexate can cause birth defects in experimental animals (see also: Phenytoin in pregnancy, page 32).[20,32,54]

Because frequent seizures pose a significant risk to the expectant mother and to the fetus as well, it is generally considered necessary for the expectant mother to continue taking her antiepileptic medication. The dosage requirements, particularly that of phenytoin, may change in some, but not all patients during pregnancy.[36,42] The phenytoin blood level may fall and the seizure frequency increase, mostly in the third trimester, necessitating an increase in dosage. This may be caused by "dilution" of the drug into a rapidly increasing volume, or by alteration of the rate of elimination, or both. After delivery, the dosage requirements decline to equal that of pre-pregnancy.

Folic acid in doses of 1 to 5 mg daily is often given during pregnancy with the intent to reduce the chances of birth defects. Whether this is effective, remains to be established by controlled prospective studies.[54]

Neonatal bleeding and clotting defects occur rarely in babies born to mothers taking antiepileptic drugs as a result of disturbed vitamin K utilization. Giving the mother vitamin K, 5 mg weekly during the last month of pregnancy, and 1 mg to the newborn seems advisable.[62]

Whether a mother who is taking antiepileptic drugs may nurse the baby, depends on her drug regimen. Phenobarbital is usually found in breast milk in concentrations of one half of that of plasma; thus, if the mother is taking high doses, the baby may receive a sedative amount. Phenytoin concentration in the breast milk, however, is about one tenth of that of plasma; thus, insignificant amounts would be received by the baby in most cases.

REFERENCES

1. BOOKER HE: Trimethadione and other oxazolidinediones. Relation of plasma levels to clinical control. In: Antiepileptic Drugs. Eds.: DM Woodbury, JK Penry, RP Schmidt. Raven Press, New York, pp 403–407, 1972.
2. BUCHTHAL F, SVENSMARK O: Serum concentration of diphenylhydantoin (phenytoin) and phenobarbital and their relation to therapeutic and toxic effects. Psychiat Neurol Neurochir 74: 117–136, 1971.
3. CHAMBERLIN HR, WADDELL WJ, BUTLER TC: A study of the product of demethylation of trimethadione in the control of petit mal epilepsy. Neurology 15: 449–454, 1965.
4. CHRISTIANSEN J, DAM M: Influence of phenobarbital and diphenylhydantoin on plasma carbamazepine levels in patients with epilepsy. Acta Neurol Scand 49: 543–546, 1973.
5. CRANFORD RE, LEPPIK IE, PATRICK B, et al: Intravenous phenytoin: clinical and pharmacokinetic aspects. Neurology 28: 874–880, 1978.
6. CUMMINGS NP, ROSENBLOOM AL, KOHLER WC, et al: Plasma glucose and insulin responses to oral glucose with chronic diphenylhydantoin therapy. Pediatrics 51: 1091–1093, 1973.
7. DALBY M: Behavioral effects of carbamazepine. In: Advances of Neurology, Vol. II. Eds: JK Penry, DD Daly. Raven Press, New York, pp 331–344, 1975.
8. EADIE MJ: Plasma level monitoring of anticonvulsants. Clin Pharmacol 1: 52–66, 1976.
9. EADIE MJ, TYRER JH: Anticonvulsant therapy. Pharmacological basis and practice. Churchill Livingstone, Edinburgh, 1974.
10. FERNGREEN HG: Diazepam treatment for acute convulsions in children. Epilepsia 15: 27–37, 1974.
11. FINCHAM RW, SCHOTTELIUS DD, SAHS AL: The influence of diphenylhydantoin on primidone metabolism. Arch Neurol 30: 259–262, 1974.
12. FRIGERIO A, MORSELLI PL: Carbamazepine: Biotransformation. In: Advances in Neurology, Vol. II. Eds. JK Penry, DD Daly. Raven Press, New York. pp 295–308, 1975.
13. GASTAUT H: Clinical and electroencephalographic classification of epileptic seizures. Epilepsia 11: 102–113, 1970.
14. GLASER GH, PENRY JK, WOODBURY DM: Antiepileptic Drugs. Mechanism of Action. Raven Press, New York (in press), 1979.

15. GLAZKO J: Antiepileptic drugs: Biotransformation, metabolism and serum half-life. Epilepsia 16: 367–391, 1975.
16. HAHN TJ: Bone complications of anticonvulsants (Review). Drugs 12: 201–211, 1976.
17. HEYMA P. LARKINS RG, PERRY-KEENE D, et al: Thyroid hormone levels and protein binding in patients on long-term diphenylhydantoin treatment. Clin Endocrinol 6: 369–376, 1977.
18. HOOPER WD, DUBETZ DK, BOCHNER F, et al: Plasma protein binding of carbamazepine. Clin Pharmacol Ther 17: 433–440, 1975.
19. HVIDBERG EF, DAM M: Clinical pharmacokinetics of anticonvulsants. Clin Pharmacokin 1: 161–188, 1976.
20. JANZ D: The teratogenic risk of antiepileptic drugs. Epilepsia 16: 159–169, 1975.
21. JENNETT B, MILLER JD, BRAAKMAN R: Epilepsy after non-missile depressed skull fracture. J Neurosurg 41: 208–215, 1974.
22. JULIEN RM, HOLLISTER RP: Carbamazepine: Mechanism of action. In: Advances in Neurology, Vol II. Eds. JK Penry, DD Daly. Raven Press, New York, pp 263–277, 1975.
23. KALLBERG N, AGURELL S, ERICSSON O, et al: Quantitation of phenobarbital and its main metabolites in human urine. Europ J Clin Pharmacol 9: 161–168, 1975.
24. KARLEN B, GARLE M, RANE A, et al: Assay of the major (4-hydroxylated) metabolites of diphenylhydantoin in human urine. Europ J Clin Pharmacol 8: 359–363, 1975.
25. KLOTZ U, ANTONIN KH, BRÜGEL H, et al: Disposition of diazepam and its metabolite desmethyldiazepam in patients with liver disease. Clin Pharmacol Ther 21: 430–436, 1977.
26. KUPFERBERG H: Quantitative estimation of diphenylhydantoin, primidone and phenobarbital in plasma by gas-liquid chromatography. Clin Chim Acta 29: 283–288, 1970.
27. KUTT H: Biochemical and genetic factors regulating dilantin metabolism in man. Ann NY Acad Sci 179: 704–722, 1971.
28. KUTT H: Mechanism of action of antiepileptic drugs. In: Handbook of Clinical Neurology, Vol. 15. Eds: PJ Vinken, GW Bruyn. North Holland Publishing Co, Amsterdam. pp 621–663, 1974.
29. KUTT H: Interactions of antiepileptic drugs. Epilepsia 16: 393–402, 1975.
30. KUTT H: Anticonvulsant blood levels in the management of epileptic patients. In: Clinical Neuropharmacology. Ed: HL Klawans. Raven Press, New York, pp 1–13, 1978.
31. KUTT H, PENRY JK: Usefulness of blood levels of antiepileptic drugs. Arch Neurol 31: 283–288, 1974.
32. KUTT H, SOLOMON GE: Relevant side effects of phenytoin. In: Antiepileptic Drugs: Mechanisms of Action: Eds: GH Glaser, JK Penry, DM Woodbury. Raven Press, New York (in press), 1979.
33. LACY JR, PENRY JK: Infantile Spasms. Raven Press, New York, 1976.
34. LAI AA, LEVY RH, CUTLER RE: Time-course of interaction between carbamazepine and clonazepam in normal man. Clin Pharmacol Ther 24: 316–323, 1978.
35. LAIDLAW J, RICHENS A: A Textbook of Epilepsy. Churchill Livingstone, Edinburgh, London and New York, 1976.

36. LANDER CM, EDWARDS VE, EADIE MJ, et al: Plasma anticonvulsant concentrations during pregnancy. Neurology 27: 128–131, 1977.
37. LENNOX-BUCHTHAL MA: Febrile convulsions: A re-appraisal. Electroencephalogr Clin Neurophysiol 32 (suppl), 1973.
38. LOUIS S, KUTT H, McDOWELL F: Intravenous diphenylhydantoin in experimental seizures. II. Effect on penicillin-induced seizures in the cat. Arch Neurol 18: 472–477, 1968.
39. LUND L: Anticonvulsant effect of diphenylhydantoin relative to plasma levels. A prospective three-year study in ambulant patients with generalized epileptic seizures. Arch Neurol 31: 289–294, 1974.
40. MAWER GE, MULLEN PW, ROGERS EM, et al: Phenytoin dose adjustment in epileptic patients. Brit J Clin Pharmacol 1: 163–168, 1974.
41. METRAKOS K, METRAKOS JD: Genetics of epilepsy. In: Handbook of Clinical Neurology, Vol 15. Eds: PJ Vinken, GW Bruyn. North Holland Publishing Co, Amsterdam. pp 429–486. 1974.
42. MYGIND KI, DAM M, CHRISTIANSEN J: Phenytoin and phenobarbital plasma clearance during pregnancy. Acta Neurol Scand 54: 160–166, 1976.
43. NICOL CF, TUTTON GC, SMITH BH: Parenteral diazepam in status epilepticus. Neurology 19: 332–343, 1969.
44. NOWACK WJ, JOHNSON RN, ENGLANDER RN, et al: Effects of valproate and ethosuximide on thalamocortical excitability. Neurology 29: 96–99, 1979.
45. ODAR-CEDERLÖF I, BORGA O: Impaired plasma protein binding of phenytoin in uremia and displacement effect of salicylic acid. Clin Pharmacol Ther 20: 36–47, 1976.
46. OXBURY JM, WHITTY CWM: Causes and consequences of status epilepticus in adults. Brain 94: 733–744, 1971.
47. PENRY JK, PORTER RJ, DREIFUSS FE: Ethosuximide. Relation of plasma levels to clinical control. In: Antiepileptic Drugs. Eds: DM Woodbury, JK Penry, RP Schmidt. Raven Press, New York. pp 431–441, 1972.
48. PINDER RM, BROGDEN RN, SPEIGHT TM, et al: Clonazepam: A review of its pharmacological properties and therapeutic efficacy in epilepsy. Drugs 12: 321–361, 1976.
49. PINDER RM, BROGDEN RN, SPEIGHT TM, et al: Sodium valproate: A review of its pharmacological properties and therapeutic efficacy in epilepsy. Drugs 13: 81–123, 1977.
50. PIPPENGER CE, PENRY JK, WHITE BG, et al: Interlaboratory variability in determination of plasma antiepileptic drug concentrations. Arch Neurol 33: 351–355, 1976.
51. PIPPENGER CE, PENRY JK, KUTT H: Antiepileptic Drugs: Quantitative Analysis and Interpretation. Raven Press, New York. 1978.
52. PORTER RJ, PENRY JK, LACY JR, et al: The clinical efficacy and pharmacokinetics of phensuximide and methsuximide. Neurology 27: 375–376, 1977.
53. RANE A, WILSON JT: Clinical pharmacokinetics in infants and children. Clin Pharmacokinet 1: 2–24, 1976.
54. REYNOLDS EH: Chronic antiepileptic toxicity. A review. Epilepsia 16: 319–352, 1975.
55. REYNOLDS EH, CHADWICK D, GALBRAITH AW: One drug (phenytoin) in the treatment of epilepsy. Lancet 2: 923–925, 1976.

56. RICHENS A: Interactions with antiepileptic drugs. Drugs 3: 266–310, 1977.

57. SCHEIBEL ME, CRANDALL PH, SCHEIBEL AB: The hippocampal dentate complex in temporal lobe epilepsy. Epilepsia 15: 55–80, 1974.

58. SCHOBBEN F, VAN DER KLEIJN E, GABREËLS F: Pharmacokinetics of di-n-propylacetate in epileptic patients. Eur J Clin Pharmacol 8: 97–102, 1975.

59. SHERWIN AL, ROBB JP, LECHTER M: Improved control of epilepsy by monitoring plasma ethosuximide. Arch Neurol 28: 178–181, 1973.

60. SIMON D, PENRY JK: Sodium di-N-propylacetate (DPA) in the treatment of epilepsy. Epilepsia 16: 549–573, 1975.

61. SIMONSEN N, OLSEN PZ, KÜHL V, et al: A comparative controlled study between carbamazepine and diphenylhydantoin in psychomotor epilepsy. Epilepsia 17: 169–176, 1976.

62. SOLOMON GE, HILGARTNER MW, KUTT H: Coagulation defects caused by diphenylhydantoin. Neurology 22: 1166–1171, 1972.

63. SOLOMON GE, PLUM F: Clinical Management of Seizures. W. B. Saunders Co, Philadelphia, 1976.

64. STRONG JM, ABEM T, GIBBS EL, et al: Plasma levels of methsuximide and N-desmethylmethsuximide during methsuximide therapy. Neurology 24: 250–255, 1974.

65. SUTTON G, KUPFERBERG HJ: Isoniazid as an inhibitor of primidone metabolism. Neurology 25: 1179–1181, 1975.

66. TROUPIN AS, OJEMANN LM, DODRILL CB: Mephenytoin: A reappraisal. Epilepsia 17: 403–414, 1976.

67. WALLIS W, KUTT H, McDOWELL F: Intravenous diphenylhydantoin in treatment of acute repetitive seizures. Neurology 18: 513–525, 1968.

68. WARD AA: The epileptic neuron: Chronic foci in animals and man. In: Basic Mechanisms of the Epilepsies. Eds: HH Jasper, AA Ward, A Pope. Little, Brown and Co, Boston. pp 263–274, 1969.

69. WILDER BJ, SCHIMPFF BD, COLLINS GH: Ultrastructure study of the chronic experimental epileptic focus. Epilepsia 13: 341–355, 1972.

70. WILDER BJ, RAMSAY RE, WILLMORE LJ, et al: Efficacy of intravenous phenytoin in the treatment of status epilepticus: kinetics of central nervous system penetration. Ann Neurol 1: 511–518, 1977.

71. WILENSKY AJ, LOWDEN JA: Inadequate serum levels after intramuscular administration of diphenylhydantoin. Neurology 23: 318–324, 1973.

72. WILSON JT, HÖJER B, RANE A: Loading and conventional dose therapy with phenytoin in children: kinetic profile of parent drug and main metabolite in plasma. Clin Pharmacol Ther 20: 48–58, 1976.

73. WOLF SM, CARR A, DAVIS DC: The value of phenobarbital in the child who has had a single seizure: a controlled prospective study. Pediatrics 59: 378–385, 1977.

74. WOODBURY DM, PENRY JK, SCHMIDT RP: Antiepileptic Drugs. Raven Press, New York, 1972.

75. ZAVADIL P. GALLAGHER BB: Metabolism and excretion of ^{14}C-primidone in epileptic patients. In: Epileptology. Ed: D Janz. Georg Thieme Publishers, Stuttgart. pp 129–139, 1976.

76. ZUCKERMAN EC, GLASER GH: Activation of experimental epileptogenic foci. Arch Neurol 23: 358–364, 1970.

3
Extrapyramidal Syndromes

Extrapyramidal diseases are classified as a group of motor disorders clinically characterized by some degree of abnormal movement, changes in the muscle tone and resistance to passive movement of the extremities, and usually some alteration in the amount of automatic movement and spontaneous movement. The group includes a variety of clinical entities such as Parkinson's disease, Sydenham's chorea, Huntington's chorea, cerebral athetosis, dystonia musculorum deformans, hemiballismus, Wilson's disease or hepatolenticular degeneration, Gilles de la Tourette's syndrome, essential or hereditary tremor and drug-induced extrapyramidal disorders associated with the use of tranquilizers such as phenothiazines. In general, extrapyramidal diseases are difficult to treat pharmacologically, and their etiology is generally poorly understood. Recently, with new developments in the understanding of neurotransmitters in the brain, their pathophysiology is becoming more clear. They will be discussed separately as treatments are generally unique to each particular disorder.

PARKINSON'S DISEASE

The diagnosis of Parkinson's disease is not difficult. Usually each patient encountered will have some degree of poverty of movement or bradykinesia (in one half of the body, or the entire body), often, some degree of rapid rhythmic tremor, (present at rest but absent during volitional activity) some degree of rigidity, (usually a cogwheel sensation of resistance in an extremity on examination) and some loss of automatic postural movements such as arm swing when walking or the ability to correct balance when the center of gravity is deviated. Less disabling symptoms include sialorrhea, seborrhea and fixed facial expression. Parkinson's disease is the most common of the extrapyramidal disorders and the most frequently encountered by a general physician. Recently, treatment has been revolutionized by use of specific substances known to be lacking in the brains of patients.

Pathophysiology

Until the early 1960's, the most striking known pathology in patients with Parkinson's disease was the loss of pigmented cells in the substantia nigra, either on one side or both sides of the brain.[23] In addition, there was often evidence of a general reduction in the cell populations in parts of the basal ganglia such as the caudate nucleus, putamen and globus pallidus, and often evidence of loss of bulk and a loss of cells in the cerebral cortex. Studies on catecholamine chemistry in the early 1960's demonstrated that the amino acid, dopamine, was an important constituent of the human brain and that it was concentrated in the substantia nigra, caudate nucleus and other parts of the extrapyramidal system.[49] This observation was made after the demonstration that reserpine, when given to experimental animals and patients, produced a Parkinson-like picture and depleted the CNS of dopamine. This state was reversed in animals by the injection of dopa and the Parkinson-like symptoms relieved.[10] Further study of the role of dopamine in the CNS has disclosed several specific neural systems which use dopamine as a neurotransmitter. These systems involve the brain stem, basal ganglia, hypothalamus, pituitary and the cerebral cortex. The system which is primarily responsible for Parkinsonism is the neural tract connecting the substantia nigra and the striatum.[1] Dopamine produced in the substantia nigra is transported along axons and released in the caudate nucleus and globus pallidus. The existence of several other dopaminergic systems in the brain suggests that Parkinson's disease may involve changes both physiologic and pathologic in more than just the substantia nigra and closely related basal ganglia.

In the early sixties, Hornykiewicz and his group in Vienna, demonstrated that in patients dying with Parkinson's disease there was a consistent reduction in the amount of dopamine in extrapyramidal structures, especially in the caudate nucleus, the substantia nigra and the globus pallidus.[27] Subsequent investigations of the content of neurotransmitters in patients with Parkinson's disease has confirmed this loss of dopamine as well as a reduction in other neurotransmitters such as serotonin, noradrenaline and probably gamma-aminobutyric acid. The decline in the concentrations of several neurotransmitters has led to the speculation that Parkinsonian symptoms might be related to an imbalance in these substances, with an alteration in the degree of inhibition and excitation in various neural systems. More sophisticated studies have demonstrated that the enzyme necessary for conversion of dihy-droxyphenylalanine (dopa) to dopamine is also reduced in the diseased areas.[35] These findings led to the logical conclusion that replacement of the dopamine loss might be beneficial for patients with Parkinson's disease. Numerous attempts were made during the early 1960's by giving small amounts of dopa to patients with Parkinson's disease either intravenously or orally.[8] Some beneficial effects were noted but no consistent improvement was observed. Cotzias, in 1966 and 1967, demonstrated that increasingly large amounts of dopa, given orally over a long period of time, produced striking and consistent improvement in the symptoms and signs of Parkinson's disease.[19] This finding has been confirmed by numerous authors since, and dopa is now believed to be the most effective treatment for patients with Parkinson's disease.[38,42,66,3] The high doses of dopa are necessary because the substance is rapidly metabolized outside the brain.

The administration of dopa is associated with a number of side effects usually having to do with the effects of high concentrations of dopamine outside the brain affecting neural systems not protected by the blood-brain barrier. The major side effects are nausea, vomiting and orthostatic hypotension. Ways were sought by which more dopa could be provided for the central nervous system while reducing the amount of peripherally circulating dopamine. A number of inhibitors of aromatic decarboxylase were known and studies were made to see if they could be used with oral dopa to reduce the peripheral metabolism of dopa. Some were found to be effective and two are now used with dopa as adjuncts to treatment.[4] The main advantage of these decarboxylase inhibitors is that they do not cross the blood-brain barrier, and do not interfere with the decarboxylation of dopa to dopamine inside the central nervous system, but virtually totally, systemically block this conversion. They have been effective in reducing the level of circulating dopamine and reducing side effects such as nausea, vomiting and hypotension.

Pharmacological interest in the problem of the dopaminergic neural system, which in Parkinson's disease is deficient, has also centered on the development of agents which could bypass the need for conversion of dopa to dopamine at the synapse and have a direct dopaminergic action on the effector cell. A number of such drugs have been discovered. These include such agents as apomorphine and its derivatives, piribedil, and certain derivatives of ergot, all of which have been tried in therapy.[58,17,9,34]

Treatment

Treatment of Parkinson's disease is entirely directed to the relief of symptoms, because there is nothing known which stops the progression of the disorder. By the time a patient with Parkinson's disease comes to the physician for help, there is usually some evidence of slowness of movement, difficulty in performing daily activities, such as dressing, bathing, eating, writing, speaking and often some obvious manifestation such as tremor. The rate of progression of the disorder prior to treatment is usually slow and this rate determines the rate of progression after treatment. Some patients, when examined initially before treatment is begun, will show some loss of higher intellectual functions, with difficulty in memory, calculation, organization, interest in social activities, and ability to be productive at work.

Often, patients will come to their physicians already treated with a number of anti-Parkinsonian agents. Formerly, the most commonly used agents for the treatment of Parkinson's disease were atropine-like drugs with an anticholinergic effect. These drugs have an antagonistic effect to acetylcholine and have been used empirically in the treatment of Parkinson's disease for over a century. Until the beneficial effect of levodopa was demonstrated, anticholinergic drugs were the main form of therapy.

The exact role of acetylcholine excess and dopamine deficiency in the genesis of Parkinson's disease is not clear. What is clear is that drugs which antagonize acetylcholine improve symptoms slightly.

The available anticholinergic drugs used have similar pharmacologic actions and beneficial effects for patients with Parkinson's disease. All have untoward side effects such as pupillary dilation, dryness of mouth, occasional urinary retention, constipation and mental confusion in common. Anticholinergic agents still have a place in the treatment of Parkinson's disease, but they are now rarely the agents with which one begins treatment. For patients who do not respond to dopa or who show less of a response than anticipated, anticholinergic agents should be tried in increasing doses until side effects become distressing or until improvement occurs. Generally, trihexyphenidyl or benztropine are the drugs most commonly used in the United States. Trihexyphenidyl is usually started in a dose of 2 mg twice a day with the dose increased gradually to 2 mg four to five times a day before discontinuing. Benztropine is somewhat more potent and should be started in a dose of 0.5 mg twice a day, increasing doses to the point where beneficial effects are observed, or side effects become noticeable requiring discontinuation of the drug. The starting and maximal doses for the commonly used anticholinergic drugs are given in Table 3-1. None of these drugs have any long term harmful effect other than producing the often complained of dryness of the mouth, blurred vision and constipation. Occasionally, the elderly male patient who has prostatism may experience acute urinary retention which always requires stopping the drug. Anticholinergic drugs often produce delirium. When evidence of a cloudy sensorium is present with poor memory, confusion and at times hallucination, anticholinergic medication should be stopped. Discontinuance of anticholinergic medications should always be considered if, (1)

Table 3-1 / Anticholinergic Drugs Commonly Used in the Treatment of Parkinson's Disease

Drug	Initial dose (mg)	Maximal dose (mg day)
Trihexyphenidyl (Artane)	1–2 twice a day	up to 20
Benztropine Mesylate (Cogentin)	.5–1 twice a day	6–8
Biperiden (Akineton)	2–4 a day	8–10
Procyclidine (Kemadrin)	5–10 a day	2–30
Cycrimine (Pagitane)	1–3 three times a day	15–20
Orphenadrine (Disipal)	50 three times a day	200–300
Chlorphenozamine (Phenoxene)	50 three times a day	200–300
Ethopropazine (Par-sidol)	10 three times a day	500–700

they are clearly not effective; (2) if the side effects such as dry mouth, blurred vision and delirium produce more distress for the patient than the symptoms of Parkinson's disease; and (3) if there is a major problem with urinary retention. Constipation is rarely an indication for stopping anticholinergic drugs, as patients with Parkinson's disease generally tend to be constipated and cessation of medication rarely improves the situation. For patients who have been taking anticholinergic medication for long periods of time, they should not be stopped abruptly prior to the initiation of any other treatment such as levodopa. Sudden stopping may produce apparent, rapid worsening of the symptoms of Parkinson's disease, often to the point that the patient becomes seriously ill from marked immobility and rigidity.[22] In some instances, fatalities have been reported from the abrupt cessation of anticholinergic medication.

Levodopa, with or without an aromatic decarboxylase inhibitor in combination, is currently the most effective available treatment for Parkinson's disease.[53] Generally, there is preference for giving levodopa with a decarboxylase inhibitor because the incidence of distressing side effects is generally reduced.

The decarboxylase inhibitor available in the United States is alpha methyl-dopa hydrazine (carbidopa) combined with dopa in ratios of 10/100 or 25/250 (inhibitor/dopa) in a tablet marketed as Sinemet. The other decarboxylase inhibitor is benserazide available with dopa in ratios of 25/100 and 50/200. Either decarboxylase inhibitor is quite effective in reducing the peripheral metabolism of levodopa and reducing the overall amount of levodopa required by the patient.

If a patient with Parkinson's disease has been previously untreated and the symptoms of Parkinson's disease do not interfere with daily life, the physician is faced with the question of whether or not to start treatment. In general, treatment should only be given when it can be expected to improve the patient's disability 20–25 percent. This means that a patient with Parkinson's disease should have experienced some trouble with daily activities such as dressing, eating, walking, etc. Patients with minimal symptoms and minimal decrease in function are probably best left untreated and periodically followed to determine the rate of progression of the disorder. Each situation must be weighed individually and physicians will often find it expedient to treat minimally involved patients.

Treatment is best started with small amounts of dopa with a decarboxylase inhibitor.[65,5] The combination should be given with the dose gradually increased to the point of maximum reduction of symptoms or to the appearance of side effects. Generally, with alpha methyldopa hydrazine given with levodopa, treatment is started with 10 mg of the decarboxylase inhibitor combined with 100 mg of dopa. The average patient requires one combination tablet three times a day as the starting dose. The dose is then increased every five to seven days by one tablet until maximum improvement occurs or side effects appear. When maximum improvement or side effects appear, the dose should be reduced slightly and maintained at that level, provided the patient is able to function well at a slightly lower dose.

Evidence of improvement following the institution of dopa with or without a decarboxylase inhibitor usually begins early, with a general sense of improved well-being experienced by the patient and evidence from family and friends that the patient "looks better or seems better."[38,53] Gradually, the patient will report improved function in activities of daily living such as dressing, walking, writing, bathing, moving about the house, getting in and out of bed, and getting in and out of chairs. These activities usually become more easily and quickly performed by the patient. The patient may also report that tremor is somewhat less. Family and friends may note that the patient starts using his face and hands for expression which had been previously absent. The average patient will show improvement with dopa and a decarboxylase inhibitor usually by the time 500 mg of dopa has been administered with 50 mg of inhibitor. Maximum improvement usually occurs on average between 1 gm to 1.25 gm of dopa administered with 100 mg to 125 mg of decarboxylase inhibitor. Table 3-2.

When levodopa is not available with a decarboxylase inhibitor, the starting dose is 250 mg of levodopa twice a day with gradually increasing doses built up slowly over a long period of time. The total daily dose should be

Table 3-2 / Treatment of Parkinson's Disease With Levodopa and Levodopa With a Decarboxylase Inhibitor

Drug	Starting Dose	Dose at Start of Improvement Average	Average Effective Dose	Dose Range
Levodopa	250–500 mg/day	2.5 gm/day	3.5–4.5 gm/day	500 mgm to 8 gms/day
Levodopa+Alpha Methyl Dopa Hydrazine (Sinemet) tablet ratio 10/100 mg decarboxylase inhibitor/dopa 25–250	10/100 three times a day	40–50/400–500 mg per day	100/1000 per day	10/100 to 200/2000 mg
Levodopa+Benserazide (Madopa) ratio 25/100 50/200 mg	25/100 three times a day	100–125/400–500 mg per day		12.5/50 mg to 500/200 mg per day

increased every four to five days by 250 mg. Preferably the medication is given after meals to reduce the chance of distressing side effects such as nausea and vomiting. In view of the fact that dopa plus a decarboxylase inhibitor is available in most parts of the world, it is rarely necessary to give dopa alone. If dopa is given alone, on average, improvement appears at a dose of approximately 2.5 gm per day.[38] The average dose that produces significant improvement is 3.5 and 4.5 gm and patients rarely require more than 4.5 gm per day. A few unusual patients will show striking improvement on minute amounts of dopa and some will require very large amounts. The range of dose is extremely wide, varying from 0.5 gm to 10 or 12 gm per day. Patients who receive dopa with a decarboxylase inhibitor rarely require more than 1.5 to 2 gm of dopa with 150 to 200 mg of decarboxylase inhibitor.

Alpha-methyldopa hydrazine and benserazide are equally effective in the production of adequate peripheral decarboxylase inhibition in humans and neither drug has been shown to have any major toxic side effect.

Side effects from dopa are relatively common but much less evident when given with a decarboxylase inhibitor. Nausea and vomiting are the most distressing and most common side effects of dopa.[38,42,66] They have been largely eliminated by the use of dopa plus decarboxylase inhibitors.[65,5] Before decarboxylase inhibitors were available this symptom was usually managed by having the patient take dopa with food, and in small doses, and even then the symptom was so distressing that some patients could not take dopa. It is now extraordinarily rare to have a patient complain of nausea and vomiting when taking dopa with a decarboxylase inhibitor, but nausea does occur and when present, the combined drugs should be given in small doses after meals.

Orthostatic hypotension is a relatively common accompaniment of dopa therapy given without decarboxylase inhibitors. It is rarely symptomatic and surprisingly, patients tolerate rather low blood pressures on medication without evidence of deleterious effects. Counteracting abnormally low blood pressure has generally been difficult, but tight stockings and the very occasional administration of vasoconstrictor agents such as ephedrine in very small doses 10–20 mg twice a day have been helpful in maintaining adequate blood pressure.

Patients who have persistent difficulty with orthostatic hypotension despite treatment, and where this symptom becomes a distressing and major problem, probably have Parkinson's symptoms in addition to a generalized degeneration of the autonomic nervous system. This syndrome described by Shy and Drager is rare and has a much poorer prognosis than uncomplicated Parkinson's disease.[50]

The side effect common to both dopa and dopa plus decarboxylase inhibitors has been the appearance of abnormal involuntary movements.[5] These have appeared early in patients who have used dopa with decarboxylase inhibitors and somewhat later in patients who have been treated with dopa alone.

They usually begin with facial grimacing or restless movements of the arms and legs. Dyskinetic movements may progress to the point where the patient is severely incapacitated. The movements are dose dependent and usually when they first appear, if the dose is slightly reduced, they disappear. The appearance of these movements has been used by some investigators to indicate the maximum amount of dopa which a patient should take. Agents such as tranquilizers or muscle relaxants which suppress these abnormal involuntary movements do so usually at the expense of return of symptoms of Parkinson's disease, and their use has no advantage over reduction of dose of regular dopa or dopa plus a decarboxylase inhibitor.

A distressing problem for patients who have been treated over a long period of time with dopa is that often the abnormal involuntary movements appear at lower and lower doses. Frequently patients are willing to tolerate abnormal involuntary movements because at the time these movements appear, patients are usually generally free of evidence of tremor or evidence of hypokinesia which interfered with their activities earlier in the course of the disease. Patients often prefer a slight degree of abnormal involuntary movement because they have found that at this point they have reached their maximum potential for function.

Another distressing side effect which has occurred with both dopa and dopa with a decarboxylase inhibitor is the development of delirium.[56] Patients with Parkinson's disease often have some evidence prior to treatment of decline in intellectual function (early dementia). In this group of patients, the administration of drugs which affect the central nervous system—including dopa and dopa with decarboxylase inhibitors—sometimes produces acute confusional states with disorientation, hallucination, illusions and delusion. These symptoms are very distressing to both the patient and the family. Such changes in intellectual function and behavior should be inquired for regularly by the physician, and if present, a dose reduction of dopa or dopa and decarboxylase inhibitor should be made. If the defects in mentation are marked, the drugs should be stopped for a few days until mental activity improves. Often, patients taking levodopa or dopa plus a decarboxylase inhibitor will report only hallucinations which are frequently benign causing no fear or anxiety and which may not require a dose reduction.

Another distressing side effect associated with long term treatment of patients with dopa and dopa with decarboxylase inhibitors has been the appearance of fluctuation in response to medication, or the "on-off" phenomenon. Patients with the "on-off" response may experience sudden cessation of the benefits of dopa with the return of many of the symptoms and signs of Parkinson's disease lasting a few minutes, an hour, or an entire day with the sudden reappearance of improvement some time later. This phenomenon has developed in over half the patients treated over a long period of time (3–5 years) and for some patients has become almost as distressing as the original disease. The "on-off" periods may occur at any time of the day and are equally common in the morning, afternoon or evening. Generally, a patient will have good periods during the day totalling four or five hours. For some patients these periods can be predicted but for many they occur randomly. Patients generally report that nothing they know of brings on these periods of lack of response and nothing clearly terminates them. Frequently, although during their "off periods" they are unable to walk or move about, they are able to use their upper extremities without difficulty and speak without problems. Treatment directed towards the alleviation of the "on-off" response to date has included smaller doses of dopa given more often and spread out over the day which produces a more stable blood level. This dose program is related to the observation that "off responses" are found with low blood levels of dopa and "on responses" with high blood levels. In addition, for those who have developed "on-off" responses on regular dopa, some improvement temporarily has been noted with the use of decarboxylase inhibitors.[57] Improvement has been found using a low protein diet which improves the intestinal absorption of dopa by decreasing competition for absorption by other amino acids. Some slight improvement in the "on-off" response has been reported with use of adjunctive agents with a dopaminergic action such as piribedil, apomorphine and bromocriptine.[9,34] To date, none of these treatments has totally alleviated the phenomenon. It is of interest that those patients treated for long periods of time who do not develop the "on-off" response have generally stable blood levels of dopa throughout the day, while those who develop the response have rapidly fluctuating levels of serum dopa over a 12 to 24 hour period.

Another distressing problem associated with the long-term treatment of Parkinson's disease has been the increasing incidence of postural instability. Patients report that they are easily pushed off balance and that they frequently fall, often seriously injuring themselves. Postural instability is generally associated with some degree of start hesitation, inability to initiate walking and/or festination of gait and shuffling. The patients usually fall immediately after arising from a chair when they are off balance; when changing direction, turning or backing up; or when reaching for an object and not being close enough to the object to reach and stabilize their center of gravity. Medications for Parkinson's disease to date have not had any effect on postural instability. Patients are at times nearly totally immobilized by the problem, but occasionally they can be educated to anticipate situations in which they are likely to fall and avoid them.

Laboratory abnormalities associated with the use of dopa and dopa plus decarboxylase inhibitors have been extremely uncommon.[33] Occasional patients have developed slight changes in serum glutamic oxaloacetic transaminase, (SGOT) but values have risen and fallen without stopping the medication. An occasional patient has been reported to have a hemolytic reaction and a positive Coombs' test. To date, there have been no serious abnormalities in liver, renal, cardiac or pulmonary function associated with long term use. Occasionally, patients on regular dopa have reported an increase in extrasystoles, but this has largely been abolished with the use of dopa plus a decarboxylase inhibitor.

With treatment using dopa plus decarboxylase inhibitors and adjunctive therapy such as anticholinergic medication, generally patients remain functional for long periods of time. There is no way of predicting in advance how long a patient will respond to levodopa and remain functional. Many patients rapidly develop the "on-off" response which can be as disabling as the Parkinson's disease. Other patients show gradual development of loss of intellectual capacity or dementia, which can be as distressing and as inhibiting to normal function as the movement disorder. Dementia is thought to be a natural consequence of Parkinson's disease and not a result of medication. Most patients on dopa retain a reasonable amount of functional mobility and ability to carry out daily activities for long periods. Their main long term problems come in the form of postural instability and declining intellectual capacity. At the start of treatment, about two thirds of patients treated will show 50 percent or more improvement in function. This ratio falls to one half of patients showing 50 percent or more improvement after 5 years of treatment and to about two fifths after 8–10 years of treatment.

Adjunctive Therapy for Parkinson's Disease

A number of new agents have been introduced in the treatment of Parkinson's disease.

Amantadine hydrochloride was developed because of its antiviral properties. It was accidentally found to have anti-Parkinson effect when given to patients to protect them from flu.[49] The exact effect of amantadine on the brain is unclear, but increased release of dopamine from nerve terminals and delayed reuptake of dopamine into terminal vessels has been postulated.

Amantadine is useful in the treatment of Parkinson's disease as it produces rather rapid benefits usually with a decrease in tremor, some relief of bradykinesia and rigidity, and improvement of function. It is only effective in about two thirds of patients and its effects may not be long lasting.[21] About half of the patients who take it notice a decline in benefit after using it for 4–6 weeks. A brief vacation from the medication often restores the beneficial effects. It may be used as the initial therapy in patients with mild or moderate disease. It is also useful as adjunctive therapy with levodopa and anticholinergic medication. Starting doses are usually 100–200 mg per day. Doses of 400 mg per day or more are rarely required and higher doses carry an increased risk of side effects.

Side effects of amantadine are generally not serious. They include livedo reticularis and ankle edema which are the most common side effects.[49,21] Restlessness, insomnia, anxiety, dizziness, blurred vision and dry mouth have all been reported by patients receiving the drug. Rare episodes of convulsions have been reported with high doses of amantadine.

Apomorphine has a strong dopaminergic activity and has been used experimentally in the treatment of Parkinson's disease.[17] Improvement has been recorded with its use. The appearance of renal failure and azotemia with chronic administration make it unacceptable for treatment.[18]

Piribedil (trivastal), a dopamine agonist, has been shown to have considerable antiparkinson effects.[58,14] Its use has been associated with a high incidence of side effects such as nausea, abnormal involuntary movements and delirium. It is not available for use in the United States and is not used extensively in other countries.

Bromocriptine is an ergot derivative with a strong dopaminergic effect.[9,34,16] It has been used in patients with "on-off" response and as a substitute for L-dopa. Although effective in doses up to 75 mg/day, its use is associated with a high incidence of side effects including confusion, hallucination, hypotension, nausea and dyskinesia.

Lergotril mesylate is another ergot derivative with considerable dopaminergic effect. It has been used experimentally for Parkinson's disease with similar effects and side effects as bromocriptine.

HEPATOLENTICULAR DEGENERATION OR WILSON'S DISEASE

Hepatolenticular degeneration or Wilson's disease is a rare inherited movement disorder whose pathophysiology is largely centered in the brain and the liver.[63] The central nervous system lesion is a degeneration of the basal ganglia and cirrhosis of the liver develops. The signs of the disease are the deposition of pigment around the limbus of the cornea and the appearance of abnormal involuntary movements like chorea and often evidence of intellectual decline. Pathophysiological investigation has found that patients with this disorder excrete large amounts of copper in their urine[41] and that a copper-containing protein, ceruloplasmin, is deficient in their blood.[48] This situation leads to a decrease in the amount of serum copper that is bound to globulin, and an increasing amount of copper bound to albumin which allows copper to be deposited in large concentrations in the liver and in the brain, especially the basal ganglia, and in the tissues of the eye.

Deposition of free copper causes damage to tissues especially the liver and the brain. In addition to the abnormal copper metabolism, an aminoaciduria,[61] usually of threonine and cystine, has been found. The underlying defect in Wilson's disease is thought to be a deficiency in the synthesis of the copper binding protein ceruloplasmin.

There is evidence that Wilson's disease is a hereditary disorder because there is a large incidence of cosanguinity among patients.[6]

Treatment

Treatment of Wilson's disease is generally aimed at decreasing the intake of dietary copper or to binding copper in the body to other agents which make it unavailable for deposition in tissues. It is difficult to reduce the overall amount of copper in the diet by food selection and yet maintain good nutrition. Potassium disulfide, which makes copper in the intestinal tract insoluble and not absorbable, has been used and is given in oral doses of up to 50 mg. These doses can reduce the amount of copper available for absorption. The most effective agents for treatment are copper chelating agents such as British antilewisite or dimercaprol[20] and penicillamine.[62,52] These drugs bind copper, which is then rapidly excreted in the urine and is unavailable for deposition in the tissues. Dimercaprol must be injected intramuscularly to be effective and is frequently associated with discomfort and abscess around the injection site. Penicillamine is the treatment of choice as it is an active chelating agent which readily binds copper and can be taken by mouth. When bound to copper, the complex is readily excreted in the urine. Patients take it daily in doses up to 4 gms for the rest of their lives. Fortunately, constant treatment has been fairly effective in reducing the progression of the disease. Penicillamine has a generally low level of toxicity but may occasionally cause fever, leukopenia and skin rashes, especially in those sensitive to penicillin.

CEREBRAL ATHETOSIS

Cerebral athetosis is a movement disorder usually associated with birth trauma, sometimes with cerebral infarction or hemorrhage or kernicterus.[12] It is most commonly encountered in infants and young adults with some degree of hemiplegia and clinically consists of writhing torsion movements involving the more proximal muscles of the extremities and of the axial muscles of the trunk. The pathophysiology is somewhat obscure, but patients who have come to autopsy have shown degeneration and fibrosis of the regions around the basal ganglia near the internal capsule, often with extensive proliferation of myelinated nerve fibers in this area.

Athetotic movements may be so severe as to totally incapacitate an individual. They may be unilateral or bilateral and greatly interfere with all daily activities. Treatment has never been very satisfactory. Recently the use of levodopa,[46] with or without the use of a decarboxylase inhibitor, has been found to reduce the amount of athetosis and improve function in patients. Levodopa is not an ideal treatment, but it is believed to be better than previous pharmacological therapy which has been largely designed to sedate patients to relieve the distressing abnormal movements, usually at the price of excessive drowsiness and lack of function. Levodopa is best given with a decarboxylase inhibitor in gradually increasing doses until improvement occurs. Initial doses are 300–400 mg of dopa with 30–40 mg of alpha-methyldopa hydrazine. Doses of more than 1000–1500 mg of dopa and 100–150 mg of decarboxylase inhibitor are rarely required. The side effects of dopa given to patients with athetosis are similar to those encountered in Parkinson's disease.

HEMIBALLISMUS

Hemiballismus is a rare disorder characterized by involuntary flail-like, often violent movements of one half of the body usually largely confined to the upper extremity. The disorder is most commonly associated with cerebrovascular disease and is most frequently seen in elderly patients who have had an infarction of the upper brain stem or regions around the thalamus. Pathophysiologic evidence suggests that the subthalamic nucleus must be involved by hemorrhage or infarction to produce this disorder. Patients who have come to autopsy with hemiballismus have had damage in or around the subthalamic nucleus. Experimentally it has been possible to produce hemiballismus in animals with lesions in the subthalamic nucleus.[11] The disorder is quite characteristic clinically. It is usually self-limiting but at times the movements are so violent that

Table 3-3 / Additional Drugs Used in the Treatment of Movement Disorders

	DOPAMINE ANTAGONISTS:	
DRUG	INITIAL DOSE (MG/DAY)	DOSE RANGE (MG/DAY)
Haloperidol	1.5	6–10
Perphenazine	6	12–32
Pimozide	2	8–16
Tetrabenazine	50	75–125
Reserpine	1	0.5–1.5

the patient becomes exhausted. The natural history is for subsidence of the movements with quiescence after a period of days' or weeks' treatment. The treatment at the moment which is most effective consists of sedation with barbiturates such as phenobarbital 30–60 mg 3–4 times daily or phenothiazines such as chlorpromazine. Doses of chlorpromazine up to 100–200 mg a day are often required to stop the movements.

DYSTONIA MUSCULORUM DEFORMANS

Dystonia musculorum deformans is a rare but extremely distressing movement disorder which is usually genetically based with a clear family history, but it sometimes occurs sporadically. Division of the clinical entity into idiopathic torsion dystonia, dystonia musculorum deformans or autosomal dominant torsion dystonia is of interest, but does not alter the therapy available.[26,43] Dystonia musculorum deformans is usually found in children or young adults with a mean age of onset around 10 years. The movements usually involve axial and proximal limb muscles. Dystonic movements vary in intensity from those just noticeable to violent incapacitating ones which may be so severe that permanent postural distortion occurs. Treatment of dystonia pharmacologically has never been very satisfactory. There are a number of agents which have been used to reduce the amount of dystonic movements, such as sedatives, muscle relaxants, tranquilizers and antiparkinson drugs. Currently, the most commonly used agents are phenothiazines, diazepam, tetrabenazine or haloperidol. Often the reduction of dystonic movements with any of these agents is produced only with major sedative side effects for the patient. Patients frequently find they would rather have the symptoms than the complications of treatment. Recently, dopa has been reported to produce some improvement in patients with dystonia.[15]

Torticollis, or wry neck, is a localized form of dystonia which is largely confined to men and occurs most commonly during the fourth decade of life. Torticollis has not been particularly amenable to pharmacological therapy. Relief of the symptom is almost always associated with marked sedation. The most effective recent treatment has been sensory tactile feedback.[32,31] With treatment, the patient learns to control his own abnormal movement. It has been successful in about half of the patients treated.

HUNTINGTON'S CHOREA

Huntington's chorea is a hereditary degenerative disorder which involves the caudate nucleus but also other basal ganglia.[32] It is characterized by abnormal involuntary movements (chorea) and a decline in intellectual capacity (dementia). Either of these symptoms may precede the other by a number of years but eventually both abnormal involuntary movements and a decline in intellectual capacity characterize the disorder. Huntington's chorea usually begins in mid-life and is clearly hereditary with an autosomal dominant form of inheritance.[31] The pathophysiology of the disorder is associated with atrophy of the brain especially marked in the neostriatum and the caudate nucleus.[37] Biochemical examination of the brains of patients who have died with Huntington's chorea recently has shown significant lowering of the levels of gamma-aminobutyric acid and glutamic acid decarboxylase.[44,7] These reduced levels are generally confined to the basal ganglia, especially the caudate nucleus. Levels of other neurotransmitters have also been reduced. Dopamine and dopamine agonists have been found to increase the involuntary movements of patients with Huntington's chorea.[29] Drugs which reduce dopaminergic activity decrease the involuntary movements and are the main form of treatment.

Treatment

Treatment of Huntington's chorea is symptomatic as there is no specific agent which will alter the progressive nature of the disorder.[13] No treatment has been shown to change the decline in intellectual capacity. Occasionally, victims who become emotionally disturbed or difficult to manage can be dealt with better if tranquilized with a phenothiazine or reserpine.[13,36] Choreic movements do not usually pose a major symptomatic problem, but when they do, they can be controlled with the administration of antidopaminergic drugs, such as haloperidol in doses of 1–10 mg per day or reserpine beginning with a dose of 0.5 to 1 mg a day, and gradually adjusting the dose until symptomatic relief is obtained. Other agents which have been reported as being useful in reducing the chorea include tetrabenazine and pimozide.[40] Despite relief of choreic movements and the calming effect of some tranquilizers in patients who are emotionally disturbed, the disorder progresses and eventually institutionalization and chronic care for an incapacitated individual are necessary.

Administration of dopa to offspring of patients with Huntington's chorea has been recommended as a means of distinguishing susceptibles, because it appears that the sensitivity to levodopa may long precede the appearance of chorea in those who have inherited the disorder.[29] The advantage of being able to identify potential victims of Huntington's chorea in advance is that it may be possible to persuade them to avoid reproduction.

SYDENHAM'S CHOREA OR INFECTIOUS CHOREA

Sydenham's chorea is now a very rare condition, virtually always associated with some evidence of rheumatic fever following a hemolytic streptococcus infection but occasionally occurring in women during pregnancy. Chorea with rheumatic fever or with pregnancy is now rarely a serious threat to the life or the function of the patient. Death from chorea is extremely uncommon and in the small number of autopsied cases a generalized nonspecific CNS inflammation has been found. Sydenham's chorea may be the only manifestation of rheumatic involvement, although it is now so uncommon to encounter active rheumatic fever that the average physician in practice would rarely, if ever, see a patient with chorea. When Sydenham's chorea is diagnosed, usually there are brief choreic movements of the face, head and neck, which may be unilateral. The condition is usually self-limiting and usually stops without treatment. When chorea becomes violent it may exhaust the victim and treatment must be given.

Treatment

Treatment is symptomatic and consists largely of sedation to reduce the choreic movements and to calm the patient. Agents which are effective include barbiturates such as 30 mg of phenobarbital 3–5 times per day, chloral hydrate 500 mg up to 5 times per day, phenothiazines and haloperidol.[59] The most useful treatment is a phenothiazine such as chlorpromazine in doses of 10 mg 3 to 4 times a day or haloperidol in doses of 3–10 mg per day.[25] If active rheumatic fever is suspected and the chorea is believed to be due to inflammation of the central nervous system, corticosteriods should be given. Prednisone is the agent of choice given in doses of 5–30 mg per day. Treatment with steroid hormones is usually given for 1–2 weeks.

ESSENTIAL TREMOR

Essential tremor is a rare but disturbing condition usually confined to older people. It has a distinct hereditary pattern and is generally slowly progressive. It is mainly manifested by intention tremor of the hands and arms, but some nodding and intention tremor of the head and trunk may be evident. Tremor is absent at rest and is made worse by an intentional activity which may become disabling for the patient. It always becomes worse under stress and fatigue and is frequently reported to be relieved by alcohol.[24]

Treatment in general has relied upon the use of sedatives, but recently it has been found that propranolol, a powerful beta-adrenergic blocking agent, will reduce essential tremor[60,64] This often requires doses of up to 130–180 mg per day. Doses are gradually built up from 20 mg 2 to 3 times a day. Propranolol should not be given to patients with cardiac disease. Glutethimide, a sedative with considerable dampening effect of brain stem reflexes, is often helpful in reducing essential tremor. Doses should begin with 250 mg twice a day and rarely exceed 500 mg three times a day. The sedative action of the drug usually decreases with long term use.

DRUG-INDUCED EXTRAPYRAMIDAL DISORDER

Symptoms of Parkinsonism such as involuntary movements (tremor), akinesia and rigidity as well as dyskinesia and motor restlessness can be caused by a variety of pharmacologic agents.

Parkinsonism with bradykinesia, rigidity and at times tremor have been observed to follow the use of drugs such as reserpine, phenothiazines, haloperidol, tetrabenazine and rarely with tricyclic antidepressants.[2] Parkinson-like symptoms following use of such drugs are more common in older patients, especially women. The appearance of drug induced Parkinsonism is related to the potency of the tranquilizing agent and is most commonly seen with the more potent phenothiazines and with haloperidol. Symptoms come on gradually and usually the patient or the patient's family report gradual but progressive appearance of slowness of movement, fixed posture and fixed facial expression. Because of the dopamine depleting effect of these causative agents observed in animals, it is believed that a similar reaction takes place in the human nervous system.

Treating drug induced Parkinson's disease is best done by stopping the causative drug. If it is desirable to speed up the periods of recovery, small amounts of levodopa and decarboxylase inhibitor (Sinemet) are useful. A dose of 400–500 mg dopa and 40–50 mg of inhibitor for one to two weeks is usually all that is needed. In rare patients Parkinson's symptoms may be permanent and require constant treatment.

DRUG INDUCED DYSKINESIA

Dyskinesia associated with drug use, usually phenothiazines, can come on acutely following initial use of the drug or may develop after long periods of use or even after stopping the causative drug.[51] The most common causative drugs are phenothiazines. The more potent the phenothiazine the more likely it is to cause dyskinesia.

The dyskinetic movements most often involve the head and neck especially, the tongue and face, but the upper and lower extremities may also be involved.

The exact cause of these movements is unclear but a number of suggestions have been made including denervation hypersensitivity of dopaminergic neurons, increased production of dopamine in nerve terminals and a possible combination of both increased production of dopamine and increased sensitivity to it. The similarity of tardive and acute dyskinesia to that seen in patients with Parkinson's disease who become intoxicated with levodopa, clearly supports the likely possibility that the dyskinesia is related to increased dopaminergic activity.

Acute dyskinetic symptoms may appear shortly after starting a phenothiazine. The movements can often be violent and alarming with marked neck retraction and jaw clenching which may resemble tetanus.

Stopping the offending drug is usually all that is needed for treatment. If the movements are violent and are exhausting the patient, they can be relieved by anticholinergic drugs given orally or intravenously. The anticholinergic drug available for intravenous use is benztropine (Cogentin) and it should be given in doses of 2 mg. Also intramuscular diphenhydramine (Benadryl) up to 5 mg is useful in stopping the movements. Oral administration of the same drug for a few days should follow the intravenous or intramuscular injection.

Late onset or tardive dyskinetic movements are more difficult to treat.[30] The movements may only come on after stopping phenothiazine therapy and they may become permanent despite treatment. The movements are most common after long term treatment with phenothiazines. They are more often encountered in older patients and they may be aggravated by the usual treatment, such as anticholinergics for acute dyskinesia. The most effective treatment is the use of drugs which block dopaminergic action at the synapse of the drugs which produce the symptoms initially.

REFERENCES

1. ANDER NE, DALSTROM A, FUXE K, et al.: Ascending monoamine neurons to the telencephalon and diencephalon. Acta Physiol Scand 67: 313, 1967.
2. AYD FJ: A survey of drug induced extrapyramidal reactions. JAMA 175: 1054, 1961.
3. BARBEAU A: L-dopa therapy in Parkinson's Disease. Can Med Assoc J 101: 791, 1969.
4. BARBEAU A, MARS H, BOTEZ MI et al: Levodopa combined with peripheral decarboxylase inhibition in Parkinson's disease. Can Med Assoc J 106:1169, 1972.
5. BARBEAU A, ROY M: Six year results of treatment with Levodopa plus benzerazide in Parkinson's disease. Neurology 26:399, 1976.
6. BEARN AG: Genetic aspects of Wilson's disease. Proc R Soc Med 52–61, 1959.
7. BIRD ED, IVERSEN LL: Huntington's Chorea: postmortem measurement of glutamic acid decarboxylase choline acetyltransferase and dopamine in basal ganglia. Brain 97:457, 1974.
8. BIRKMAYER W, HORNYKIEWICZ O: Der 1,3,4 dihydroxyphenylaline (dopa) effect bei der Parkinson-Akinese. [Wien.] Klin Wochenschr. 73:787, 1961.
9. CALNE DB, TEYCHENNE PF, CLAVERIA E et al: Bromocriptine in Parkinsonism Brit Med J 4:442, 1974.
10. CARLSSON A, LINDQUIST M and MAGNUSSON T: 3,4 Dihydroxyphenylalanine and 5 hydroxytryptophane as reserpine antagonists. Nature p. 180, 1957.
11. CARPENTER MB: Ballism associated with partial destruction of the subthalamic nucleus of Luys. Neurology 5: 479, 1955.

12. CARPENTER MD: Athetosis and the basal ganglia. Arch Neurol Psychiatry 63: 875, 1950.

13. CHASE TN: Rational approaches to the pharmacotherapy of chorea in Yahr MD (ed) Basal Ganglia. New York Raven Press 1976, p 337.

14. CHASE TN, WOODS AC, GLAUBIGER GA: Parkinson's disease treated with a suspected dopamine receptor agonist. Arch Neurol 30: 383, 1974.

15. COLEMAN M: Preliminary remarks on the L-dopa therapy of dystonia. Neurology 20: 114, 1970.

16. CORRODI H, FUXE K, HOKFELT T, et al: Effect of ergot drugs on central catecholamine neurons: Evidence for a stimulation of central dopamine neurons. J Pharm Pharmacol 25: 409, 1973.

17. COTZIAS GC, LAWRENCE WH, PAPAVASILIOU PS et al: Apomorphine and Parkinsonism. Trans. Am. Neurol. Assoc. 97: 156, 1972.

18. COTZIAS GC, PAPAVASILIOU PS, TOLOSA ES et al: Treatment of Parkinson's disease with apomorphines. N Engl J Med 294: 567, 1976.

19. COTZIAS GC, VAN WOERT MH, SCHIFFA LM: Aromatic amino acids and modification of Parkinsonism. N Engl J Med 276:374, 1967.

20. DENNY-BROWN D, PORTER H: The effect of BAL (2,3-dimercaptopropanol) on hepatolenticular degeneration (Wilson's Disease). N Engl J Med 245:917, 1951.

21. FAHN S, ISGREEN WP: Long term evaluation of amantadine and levodopa combination in Parkinsonism by double-blind study. Neurology 25:695, 1975.

22. GRANGER M: Exacerbations in Parkinsonism, Neurology 2:538, 1961.

23. GREENFIELD JG and BOSANQUET FD: The brainstem lesions in Parkinsonism. J Neurol, Neurosurg Psychiatry 16:213, 1953.

24. GROWDON JH, BHAGWAN TS, YOUNG RR: Effect of alcohol on essential tremor. Neurology 25: 259, 1975.

25. HEILMAN K, KOHLER WC and LEMASTER PC: Haloperidol treatment of chorea associated with systemic lupus erythematosus. Neurology 21: 963, 1971.

26. HERZ E: Dystonia I. Historical Review II. Clinical classification III. Pathology and conclusions Arch Neurol Psychiatry 52: pp. 305, 319, 320, 1944.

27. HORNYKIEWICZ O: Metabolism of brain dopamine in human Parkinsonism, neurochemical and clinical aspects. eds. Costa E, Cote LJ and Yahr MD Biochemistry and Pharmacology of the basal ganglia. New York Raven Press 1966, p. 171.

28. HUNTINGTON G: On chorea Med Surg Reporter 26:317, 1892.

29. KLAWANS HL, PAULSON GW, RINGEL SP: Use of L-dopa in the detection of presymptomatic Huntington's Chorea. N Engl J Med 285: 1332, 1972.

30. KOBAYASHI R: Drug therapy of tardive dyskinesia. N Engl J Med 296: 257, 1977.

31. KOREIN J, BRUNDY J: Integrated EMG feedback in the management of spasmodic torticollis and focal dystonia. A prospective study of 80 patients. in Yahr MD (ed) Basal Ganglia New York Raven Press, 1976.

32. KOREIN J, BRUNDY J, GRYNBAUM B, et al: Sensory feedback therapy of spasmodic torticollis and dystonia. Results of treatment of 55 patients. Adv Neurol 14:375, 1976.

33. LANGRALL HM, JOSEPH C: Evaluation of safety and efficacy of L-Dopa in Parkinson's disease and syndrome. Neurology 22 (Suppl.): 3, 1972.

34. LIEBERMAN A, ZOLFAGHI M, BOAL D, et al: The antiparkinson efficacy of bromocriptine. Neurology 25: 405, 1976.
35. LLOYD K, HORNYKIEWICZ O: Parkinson's Disease, activity of L-Dopa decarboxylase in discrete brain regions. Science 170:, 1212 1970.
36. LYON RL: Drug treatment of Huntington's Chorea. Brit Med J 1:1308, 1962.
37. McCAUGHEY WT: The pathologica spectrum of Huntington's Chorea. J. Nerv. Ment. Dis. 133: 91, 1961.
38. McDOWELL FH, LEE JE, SWIFT T et al: Treatment of Parkinson's syndrome with L-dihyroxyphenylalanine (Levodopa) Ann. Int. Med. 72: 29, 1970.
39. McDOWELL FH, SWEET RD: The on-off phenomenon in Advances in Parkinsonism. Birkmayer, W and Hornykiewicz, O (ed) Editiones Roche Basel 1976, p. 603.
40. McLELLAN DL, CHALMERS RJ, JOHNSON RH: A double blind trial of tetrabenazine, thiopropazate and placebo in patients with chorea. Lancet 1:104, 1974.
41. MANDELBROTE BM, STAINER MW, THOMPSON RHS, THURSTON MN: Studies on copper metabolism in demyelinating diseases of the central nervous system. Brain 71: 212, 1948.
42. MARKHAM CH, TRECIOKAS LJ, DIAMOND SG: Parkinson's Disease and Levodopa. West. J. Med. 121: 188, 1974.
43. MARSDEN CD: Dystonia—The spectrum of the disease. in: Yahr MD (ed) The Basal Ganglia. New York, Raven Press, 1976.
44. PERRY TL, HANSEN S, KLOSTER M: Huntington's Chorea, deficiency of gamma-aminobutyric acid in brain. N. Engl. J. Med 288:337, 1973.
45. PRATT RTC: The Genetics of Neurological Disorders. London Oxford Univ Press, 1967.
46. ROSENTHAL RK, McDOWELL FH, COOPER W: Levodopa therapy in athetoid cerebral palsy. Neurology 22:1, 1972.
47. SANO I, GAMO T, KAMINOTO Y et al: Distribution of catechol compounds in human brain. Biochem. Biophys. Acta 32:586, 1959.
48. SCHEINBERG IH, GITLINE D: Deficiency of ceruloplasmin in patients with hepato-lenticular degeneration. Science 116:484, 1952.
49. SCHWAB RS, ENGLAND AC, JR., POSKANZER DC et al: Amantadine in the treatment of Parkinson's Disease. JAMA 208: 1168, 1969.
50. SHY GM, DRAGER CA: A Neurological syndrome associated with orthostatic hypotension. A clinical pathological study. Arch. Neurol. 2:511, 1960.
51. SIMPSON GM, KLINE NS: Tardive dyskinesia - manifestations, incidence, etiology and treatment. in: Yahr, M.D. (ed) Basal Ganglia New York Raven Press, 1976 p. 427.
52. STERNLIEB I, SCHEINBERG IH: Penicillamine therapy for hepatolenticular degeneration. JAMA 189: 748, 1964.
53. SWEET RD, McDOWELL FH: Five years treatment of Parkinsonism with L-dopa, therapeutic results and survival in 100 patients. Ann Int Med 83: 456, 1975.
54. SWEET RD, McDOWELL FH: The on-off response in chronic L-dopa treatment of Parkinsonism. in McDowell FH and Barbeau A (eds) Advances in Neurology New York, Raven Press, 1974. Vol. 5 p. 331
55. SWEET RD, McDOWELL FH: Plasma dopa levels in the on-off effect in Parkinson's Disease. Neurology 24:953, 1974.

56. Sweet RD, McDowell FH, Fiegenson JS et al: Mental symptoms in Parkinson's Disease during chronic treatment with Levodopa. Neurol. 26: 305, 1976.

57. Sweet RD, McDowell FH, Wasterlain CG, Stern PH: Treatment of the on-off effect with a dopa decarboxylase inhibitor. Arch. Neurol. 32: 560, 1975.

58. Sweet RD, Wasterlain CG, McDowell FH: Piribedil, a dopamine agonist in Parkinson's Disease. Clinical Pharmacol Ther 16:1077, 1974.

59. Tierney RC, Kaplan S: Treatment of Sydenham's Chorea. Am. J. Dis. Child. 109: 408, 1965.

60. Tolosa ES, Loewenson RC: Essential tremor treatment with propranolol. Neurology 25:1041, 1975.

61. Uzman L, Denny-Brown D: Amino aciduria in hepatolenticular degeneration. Am J Med Scien 215:599, 1948.

62. Walshe JM: Penicillamine, a new oral therapy for Wilson's Disease. Am. J. Med. 21:487, 1956.

63. Wilson SAK: Progressive lenticular degeneration. A familial nervous disease associated with cirrhosis of the liver. Brain 34: 295, 1911.

64. Winkler GF, Young RR: Efficacy of chronic propranolol therapy in action tremors of familial, senile or essential varieties. N. Engl. J. Med. 290: 984, 1974.

65. Yahr MD, Duvoisin RC, Mendoza MR et al: Modification of L-dopa therapy of Parkinsonism by alpha methyldopa hydrazine. Trans Am Neurol Assoc 96: 55, 1971.

66. Yahr MD, Duvoisin RC, Schear MJ et al: Treatment of Parkinsonism with Levodopa. Arch Neurol 21: 343, 1969.

FURTHER READING

Barbeau, A, Chase, T N and Paulson, G W (eds): Advances in Neurology: Huntington's Chorea. Raven Press, New York, 1973.

Barbeau, A and McDowell, F H (eds): L-Dopa and Parkinsonism. F A Davis, Philadelphia 1970.

Bianchine, J D, and Shaw, G M: Clinical pharmacokinetics of Levodopa in Parkinson's disease. Clinical Pharmacokinetics, 1: 313–338, 1976.

Birkmayer, W, Hornykiewicz, O (eds): Advances in Parkinsonism. Editiones Roche, Basle, 1976.

Calne, D B: Developments in the pharmacology and therapeutics of parkinsonism. Ann Neurology, 1: 111–119, 1977.

Eldridge, R and Fahn, A (eds): Advances in Neurology: Dystonia. Raven Press, New York, 1973.

Walshe, J M and Cumings, J N: Wilson's Disease. Chas C Thomas, Springfield, 1961.

Yahr, M D (ed): The Basal Ganglia. Research Publications: Assoc for Research in Nervous and Mental Disease. Vol 55. Raven Press, New York 1976.

4

Cerebrovascular Diseases

INTRODUCTION AND GENERAL PRINCIPLES

Cerebrovascular disease is perhaps the most common neurological problem that physicians are called upon to treat. Unfortunately, it is also the most devastating of neurological illnesses. In developed countries cerebrovascular diseases of all types are common, and occur more often in older patients, and in those with evidence of generalized atherosclerotic vascular disease. There are two fundamental types of cerebrovascular disease; one involving infarction of the brain and the other involving hemorrhage into or around the brain. Cerebral infarction is the most common of all cerebrovascular diseases and is most frequently associated with atherosclerotic vascular disease. Other causes of cerebral infarction include cerebral emboli from such sources as the wall of the heart, the valves of the heart, atherosclerotic plaques in arteries leading to the brain, inflammatory vascular disease involving the arteries of the brain and those leading to it, and occasionally trauma which may damage the vessels in the neck leading to the brain.

The most common cause of hemorrhage in the brain is ruptured cerebral aneurysm. Other causes of intracranial or cerebral hemorrhage include hypertension, arteriovenous anomalies, inflammation of arterial walls with the development of mycotic aneurysms and occasionally hemorrhage into neoplasms.

Because atherosclerosis is the common denominator of cerebral infarction, it is important to understand some of the features of the development of this disorder. It is most common among the populations of the well developed countries of the world, especially in those areas where high caloric, high saturated fat diets are common. It is estimated that in these countries atherosclerosis is probably present in about 95 percent of the population who reach the age of 80.[19] Atherosclerosis can often first be detected in infancy or childhood with the development of fatty streaks in the aorta. Generally, in the late teens there is evidence of atherosclerosis in the aorta and beginning evidence of atherosclerotic disease occasionally in other vessels. By the twenties and thirties atherosclerosis is commonly present in the coronary arteries and beginning to be found in the arteries leading to the brain. By the forties and fifties atherosclerosis becomes well advanced in most arterial sites including these vessels going to the brain. The problem with atherosclerosis is that it is a disorder with a long development time and complications from it do not occur until 30–40 years after its beginning. The most common complications are myocardial infarction, infarction of the brain and infarction of the extremities. In the brain, the most common sequence of events leading to infarction is atherosclerotic involvement of the arteries leading to the brain in the neck, especially the internal carotid artery at its bifurcation and in the larger arteries around the circle of Willis. The atherosclerotic process eventually leads to scarring and atherosclerotic plaque formation which may totally occlude the arteries. Occlusion is usually followed by infarction in the brain tissue supplied by a particular vessel, but also the atherosclerotic plaque may ulcerate and become a source of cerebral emboli. Regardless of the cause of cerebral infarction, whether it is due to vascular occlusion by the atherosclerotic process, embolization from structures such as heart valve, myocardial wall or the surface debris on arteries leading to the head, the results are generally the same. Brain tissue made ischemic, if it remains so for longer than 15 minutes, shows evidence of a death of nerve cells (infarction) in the ischemic area which may progress to total loss of nerve cells in the area and ultimately cystic formation. If the infarction is small it may go clinically undetected. If it is large it may produce devastating neurological problems for patients such as hemiplegia, aphasia, hemisensory loss, and hemianopsia. The metabolic demands of the brain are such that it is not capable of withstanding ischemia or loss of substrates such as oxygen or glucose for more than a few minutes. Once nerve cell degeneration is produced by loss of substrate it is unlikely that restoration of substrate will produce return of function in dead or dying nerve cells. Some marginally ischemic cells around infarcted tissue may resume a degree of normal function, but the cells in the center of the infarcted area, despite any known measures, cannot be restored to life or function. A number of promising experimental approaches to the problem have been made, showing that nerve tissue exposed to relatively high concentrations of barbiturates and certain anesthetics prior to the introduction of ischemia will remain viable when ischemic for longer periods of time.[32] This has not yet been applicable to the human situation because one usually encounters clinical evidence of brain ischemia only after it is beyond the point of reversal. In view of the fact that very little, if anything, can be done about infarcted brain, except to tide the patient over during the period of acute illness and hope that he may experience spontaneous restoration of function in marginally damaged or only partially ischemic tissue, prevention assumes the major role in therapy. Because it is possible to cause infarction in a number of ways in addition to atherosclerosis, all of these must be considered when approaching therapy prophylactically. Infarction may be caused by atherosclerotic disease of the cerebral vessel, by disorders of the heart with cardiac failure, cardiac dysrhythmia, disorders of heart valve function due to rheumatic heart disease, inflammation of heart valves and myocardial walls such as subacute bacterial endocarditis and disorders of the blood itself, such as anemia and polycythemia, or abnormalities of platelet function.[22]

Immediate treatment of an individual who is suspected of having cerebral ischemia or infarction should include careful screening for the presence of heart disease and, if evident, this should be carefully evaluated and treated. Patients should also be carefully screened and evaluated for disturbance in red cell or platelet function, and if these disorders are found they should be treated by appropriate measures.[22] Usually these conditions are not an important cause of cerebral infarction. For the individual who has developed an acute cerebrovascular accident, immediate treatment is directed toward management of life threatening conditions that may accompany a stroke. These include the problems associated with depressed states of consciousness such as maintenance of an open clear airway, treatment of possible myocardial infarction or congestive heart failure. The incidence of heart disease among patients with stroke is high and is often a major cause of disability and death. Careful management of cardiac disease is often as important to the patient as the management of his stroke. Cardiac dysrhythmia, when present, should be carefully treated as some cardiac dysrhythmias may produce enough reduction in cerebral blood flow to further increase brain ischemia. When patients are unable to take fluid and food by mouth they must be fed intravenously for brief periods. Electrolyte imbalance should be avoided. Patients unable to urinate are best treated initially by intermittent sterile catheterization rather than by indwelling catheters or parasympathetic agents.

When patients with stroke have increasing depression of levels of consciousness following the onset of the stroke, the cause is usually cerebral edema. Some cerebral edema accompanies all cerebral infarction or hemorrhages. The presence of edema usually does not become symptomatic and is rarely life threatening unless the infarct or hemorrhage is large. When vital functions are threatened by cerebral edema, transient relief may be obtained by intravenous mannitol given in doses of 50–200 gm over a period of 21–24 hours.[15] The benefits are transient and rebound phenomena may occur. Shrinking brain volume by hyperventilation and reduction of cerebral blood flow is rarely helpful in the edema from cerebral infarction.

TRANSIENT ISCHEMIC ATTACK

Many patients prior to the development of cerebral infarction often have warnings characterized by brief periods of cerebral ischemia. These brief periods are called transient ischemic attacks and their evaluation and treatment is one of the most effective means by which cerebral infarction can be prevented. Transient ischemic attacks are usually brief periods of neurologic dysfunction lasting less than 30 minutes to one hour in most cases, but sometimes continue for as long as 24 hours. The most common symptoms are weakness on one side of the body, arm and face or sensory disturbances on one side of the body or difficulty in speaking or understanding speech. Transient symptoms such as these usually come from ischemia in the brain supplied by the carotid artery. Symptoms produced by ischemia in those parts of the brain supplied by the vertebral artery include double vision, loss of vision, difficulty with facial movements, ataxia or loss of strength in both lower and upper extremities. When present, transient ischemic attacks generally indicate that for brief periods certain portions of the brain have become ischemic.

There are several causes of transient ischemic attacks. The most common probably being the flooding of the cerebral circulation by small emboli from ulcerated atherosclerotic plaques in the carotid arteries. Other causes include changes in cerebral blood flow across marked degrees of obstruction in arteries leading to the brain. Others are associated occasionally with disorders in cardiac rhythm.

Once patients have been identified as having transient ischemic attacks they should be carefully evaluated for the possibility that preventive therapy will avoid cerebral infarction. A number of current therapies are available. The potentially most effective is surgical correction of atherosclerotic arterial obstructive lesions or removal of atherosclerotic plaques. This can be accomplished only after careful angiographic evaluation of the vessels leading to the brain and around the brain, clearly identifies the presence and sites of such lesions. Surgical therapy with removal of such obstructions or plaques has been found to be most effective in those patients who have isolated areas of atherosclerosis in the internal carotid artery just beyond its bifurcation.[10,35,6,7] Patients with such lesions represent a relatively small percentage of the total problem. Often there is evidence of atherosclerosis in many other sites, including intracranial sites that are usually beyond effective surgical treatment. Extracranial intracranial anastomosis through the temporal artery-middle cerebral artery interconnection by-passing the obstruction has been used for the treatment of such patients.

For those patients not treatable by surgery it has been shown that anticoagulation and agents which reduce the tendency for platelets to adhere to one another, effectively decrease the number of transient ischemic attacks in patients who have them and probably reduce the chances of developing cerebral infarction in the future. Transient ischemic attacks occur in about one half the patients who ultimately have stroke, when questioned retrospectively; but only 10–20 percent of patients present them prior to infarction. The natural history of transient cerebral ischemia indicates that approximately one-third of patients will spontaneously stop having such attacks and not necessarily go on to have a cerebral infarction. Other patients continue having them frequently and when followed do not develop a cerebral infarction, and some patients develop infarction within hours or days after the start of these attacks. It has been shown that anticoagulation with a coumarin anticoagulant, sometimes beginning with heparin, effectively reduces the frequency of transient ischemic attacks and the evidence, although not ideal, suggests that patients continued on anticoagulation with coumarin anticoagulants have less chance of developing stroke in the future. Patients given anticoagulants after the diagnostic evaluation has been made, are maintained with prothrombin times of approximately one and a half to two times the control value.[27,12] Management of patients on anticoagulants is not difficult if a number of considerations are kept in mind. First of all, it is important to have the total cooperation of the patient so that he takes his anticoagulants regularly, reports to his physician regularly for evaluation of his prothrombin time, reports other illnesses or other medications he may be receiving from other physicians and intelligently understands the potential complications of anticoagulants. Warfarin sodium (Coumadin) is the most commonly used anticoagulant. Daily doses vary depending on the prothrombin time. Enough is given to keep the prothrombin time at about two times normal. Induction of anticoagulation is done with a large initial dose of 30–50 mg, then usually followed by a maintenance dose of 2–10 mg per day. Prothrombin times are measured daily until the level reaches the desired range often enough to be certain that a given dose produces a desired response. Treatment for over-dosage or excessive prothrombin times is done with vitamin K. Usually, oral doses of up to 10 mg are sufficient but occasionally parenteral vitamin K in doses up to 25 mg must be given. Vitamin K resistant changes in prothombin times must be treated with transfusion. Patients with transient ischemic attacks are generally kept on anticoagulants for three to six months.[33,21,14] The drugs are then reduced and stopped but reinstituted if the patient develops further symptoms. Anticoagulation of patients is totally contraindicated if there is a suggestion of bleeding into the spinal fluid or if there is a previous history of bleeding peptic ulcer. Patients with sustained hypertension should not receive anticoagulants, but if their hypertension is well controlled and their transient ischemic problems are serious enough, they may be considered for anticoagulants. Once a patient's response to a given dose of Coumadin has been established it is possible for patients to be followed as infrequently as once a month or once every two months with prothrombin times, providing the patients are aware of the difficulties associated with anticoagulants. They must report to their physicians any untoward experiences or report before any surgical procedure, or tooth extraction is undertaken. Patients who take anticoagulants over long periods of time must be careful about their diets, avoiding situations in which large amounts of vitamin K are consumed and they must be very careful about taking other agents such as aspirin which alter platelet function and increase the chance of hemorrhage.[14] Patients who do bleed while on anticoagulants should be carefully evaluated as there is often an underlying reason for their bleeding. Gastrointestinal bleeding often signals development of occult malignancy, bleeding in the urinary tract should also signal an evaluation for the potential of a bleeding source not related to the original problem of cerebral ischemia.[41]

It has recently been demonstrated that some patients with thrombocythemia have a high frequency of transient ischemic attacks.[24] In those patients with excessive platelets, agents which reduce the chances of platelets adhering to one another or adhering to the intimal surface of vessels have been shown to reduce the frequency of transient ischemic attacks.[8] The agents that are generally used are acetylsalicylic acid (aspirin), dipyridamole and sulfinpyrazone. Combinations of these drugs have been recommended. Perhaps the safest and most frequently used agent is aspirin. Drugs which reduce platelet adherence have been used for patients with transient ischemic attacks who do not have excessive platelets and evidence has accumulated from a national cooperative study in the United States and from studies elsewhere that aspirin, if taken regularly in quantities of 1200–1800 mg a day, will effectively reduce platelet adherence and reduce the frequency of transient ischemic attacks. Studies to date have shown that such treatment reduced the future chances of cerebral infarction and death in males, not in females.[9,2] Aspirin and sulfinpyrazone are now widely used for the treatment of transient ischemic attacks and they are the treatment of choice for men who are not good candidates for vascular surgery.

Patients who do have transient ischemic attacks should also be carefully medically evaluated. If hypertension is present, this should be treated, if they are obese, their weight should be reduced, if they smoke they should be encouraged to discontinue smoking. All of these situations seem to enhance the chances of developing stroke. The frequency of transient ischemic attacks and stroke rises with increasing age; the most common age group in which they are encountered are from 60 to 80; however, young persons occasionally will develop such symptoms and it is not infrequent that young women taking contraceptive medication will have symptoms of cerebral ischemia and stroke.

PROGRESSING STROKE

Occasionally a physician encounters a patient who is showing clinical evidence of cerebral ischemia and during a relatively brief period, while under observation, shows progressing neurological dysfunction suggesting increasing cerebral infarction. Such a situation is called progressing stroke and calls for immediate and urgent treatment.[36,1] It is often difficult to be sure that a stroke is progressing and, when in doubt, it is probably best to treat such patients rather than wait until they develop increasing amounts of neurologic dysfunction. The situation which has the worst prognosis and is most frightening involves evidence of ischemia of the brain stem.[40] The most effective means of stopping a progressing stroke is the use of anticoagulants.[3,21,40] When the diagnosis is made, patients should immediately be placed on heparin, approximately 15,000 units every 4–5 hours to keep the clotting time indefinitely prolonged. Patients should be continued on this regimen for approximately 5 to 7 days. At the same time heparin is started, coumarin anticoagulants should be started. Once the prothrombin time reaches two to two and a half times normal control, generally heparin can be discontinued. Coumarin anticoagulants should then be continued for three to six months once the patient shows evidence of stabilized neurological function. In rare instances patients will not respond to this regimen. When this occurs, they should be carefully screened for the possibility that the cause of the progressing infarction is multiple cerebral emboli arising from atherosclerotic plaques in the carotid artery. In such situations, platelet anti-adherent agents such as aspirin should be added to the medical regimen, and if this does not stop the transient ischemic attacks, surgical intervention with removal of ulcerated plaque or obstructive atherosclerotic plaque should be undertaken immediately.

Agents which produce cerebral vasodilatation or change the characteristics of flow in cerebral arteries have not been shown to clearly affect the outcome of patients with stroke. A number of such treatments have been tried including the inhalation of carbon dioxide, the use of papaverine, and the use of glycerol.

Most areas of cerebral infarction are accompanied by some degree of cerebral swelling. If the infarction is very large, cerebral swelling with brain edema and shift of brain substance may threaten the life of the patients. Because of this, a number of agents have been tried to reduce cerebral edema. These include agents such as hypertonic urea solutions, mannitol, glycerol and corticosteroids.[16] None of these agents has been shown to effectively reduce cerebral edema and none in clinical trials have been shown to alter the outcome of patients with stroke and cerebral edema. During periods following infarction when cerebral edema is present it usually reaches its maximum within one to three days after infarction and persists for three or four days. When this occurs, the patient should be carefully nursed with vital functions being persevered as well as possible to tide the patient through the period of greatest danger. Measures include maintenance of open airways, careful tracheal and bronchial toilette, artificial ventilation if necessary, fluid and food intravenously or by gastric tube and careful attention to the skin for development of pressure sores.

Following recovery from the acute phases of infarction, patients should be immediately started on programs of active and passive exercises for rehabilitation and reeducation of remaining function. This is most effective if started early, generally within one to two days after the patient has stabilized following cerebral infarction. This treatment should continue throughout the remaining life of the patient. It is important that all muscles be fully stretched and all joints fully ranged several times a day to prevent joint constriction and muscle and tendon shortening. Patients even with devastating amounts of loss of neural function can often be educated to effectively take care of themselves and to retain some degree of independence following cerebral infarction. Fortunately, not all cerebral infarctions are catastrophic and many patients are, despite their disabilities, able to continue active and productive lives.

CEREBRAL EMBOLI

For patients who develop cerebral infarction with cerebral emboli from the heart, rheumatic heart disease with mitral stenosis and auricular fibrillation is the most common cause.[18] Other causes of cerebral emboli are myocardial infarction with emboli from thrombi forming on infarcted intracardiac intimal surface. Such emboli are usually multiple and patients who develop a sudden onset of neurological dysfunction following or associated with myocardial infarction or are known to have rheumatic heart disease, especially with mitral stenosis and auricular fibrillation, should be immediately placed on anticoagulants.[42,17] Usually this is accomplished by immediately starting coumarin anticoagulation and continuing the patient on this treatment indefinitely if he has rheumatic heart disease and for several months following a myocardial infarction. The use of anticoagulants in patients with rheumatic heart disease has been clearly shown to definitively reduce the chances of recurrent cerebral emboli and infarction and reduce the morbidity and mortality from cerebral emboli.[38,4,5] When present, mitral stenosis should be corrected surgically, if applicable, but even after this is done the patient should be continued on anticoagulation. For patients with auricular fibrillation, conversion to normal rhythm is sometimes useful, but patients who have mitral stenosis have been found to develop cerebral emboli even during periods of normal sinus rhythm.

Anticoagulants do not provide perfect protection against the possible development of cerebral infarction as patients who are fully anticoagulated occasionally will develop a cerebral embolus.[39] Patients with inflammatory arteritis should be treated for the basic underlying process. Usually the most frequent cause is periarteritis and occasionally lupus erythematosus. In both instances treatment with steroids is beneficial.

SUBARACHNOID HEMORRHAGE

The most common cause of nontraumatic intracranial hemorrhage is ruptured berry aneurysm.[30] In view of the fact that aneurysms are rarely evident until they rupture, producing subarachnoid hemorrhage with or without intracerebral extension, there is no way to anticipate their presence. Occasionally, cerebral aneurysms will become large enough so that they produce symptoms and signs similar to those of a brain tumor. In such instances, aneurysm is usually diagnosed after angiogram, not before, and only presumption of an expanding intracranial mass of unknown cause can be made prior to the angiogram.

In patients who develop subarachnoid hemorrhage, with or without intracerebral extension of the bleeding, the problem is extremely serious as there is a high mortality and high morbidity associated with each hemorrhage; and recurrences are quite common.[30] Prevention of recurrences is the major goal of therapy. Efforts at preventing recurrences are directed largely at surgical removal of the aneurysm or reinforcement of aneurysmal wall. This is variably effective. Most patients cannot generally tolerate the stress of surgery until 7 to 10 days after the development of subarachnoid hemorrhage and recurrences of bleeding are most common during this period. Efforts to reduce the chances of recurrent bleeding have been directed to a number of areas. It has been observed that those patients who are hypertensive tend to have a greater chance of recurrent bleeding. Reduction of blood pressure to normal or subnormal levels has been advocated as a means of reducing further occurrences. This is difficult therapy to manage, because often, by the time effective antihypertensive treatment can be induced, bleeding has begun again. It is important in those patients with subarachnoid hemorrhage and ruptured aneurysm who are hypertensive, to bring their blood pressure, as quickly as possible, to as normal a level as possible. This can be done by a variety of means, usually reserpine or alpha methyldopa are effective. Methyldopa can be given orally 250 mg 2–4 times daily or intravenously, 500 to 1,000 mg by infusion. Reserpine is usually given intramuscularly in doses of 1–4 mg. It is rarely necessary to use more strenuous means of blood pressure reduction such as sodium nitroprusside. Blood pressure, once it is returned to normal, should be kept there and the patient continuously treated.

The meningeal irritation which follows bleeding into the subarachnoid space causes a marked enhancement of fibrinolytic activity. It is believed that this increased fibrinolytic activity may be responsible for the dissolution of clots plugging a bleeding aneurysm and may be the cause of recurrent bleeding. In view of this, recent attempts have been made to use agents which reduce fibrinolysis.[23,25,26,28] These agents include epsilon aminocaproic acid and tranexamic acid. These drugs have been given to patients with subarachnoid hemorrhage and attempts have been made to evaluate them in the United States and other countries to determine their effectiveness in reducing recurrent subarachnoid hemorrhage. There is some evidence that the use of large amounts of up to 30–40 gm of epsilon aminocaproic acid per day may reduce the chance of rebleeding following subarachnoid hemorrhage. Amounts needed are large and the treatment must be continued for at least 10 to 14 days following hemorrhage. The effectiveness of these agents is not clear enough to justify their routine use in all patients with subarachnoid hemorrhage, regardless of cause. Medical treatment at best is designed to tide the patient over critical periods of illness, to reduce high blood pressure which may enhance the chances of rebleeding, to reduce physical activity which is believed to be associated with rebleeding and to maintain the patient's nutritional, fluid and electrolyte status while he recovers from the initial insult. The mortality of this condition remains extremely high and is believed to be somewhere around 45–50 percent for each bleeding, and recurrent bleeding takes place in as many as one-third to one-half of patients.

PRIMARY INTRACEREBRAL HEMORRHAGE

Primary intracerebral hemorrhage is a relatively rare disorder and virtually universally associated with marked hypertension.[13] The pathophysiology of this condition is believed to be related to the rupture of small microaneurysms on the intracerebral vascular tree, such structures are found mainly on the branches of the lenticulostriate arteries. Charcot and Bouchard described these microscopic aneurysmal weakenings of the walls of vessels in patients who had developed intracerebral hemorrhage. Usually, however, the hemorrhage is so destructive that evidence of its cause rarely remains. Aneurysms similar to those described by Charcot and Bouchard have been produced experimentally in hypertensive rabbits and these aneurysms have been associated with a high incidence of primary intracerebral hemorrhage in these animals.[31]

Intracerebral hemorrhage is most often confined to the center of the brain in the region of the basal ganglia and the internal capsule. However, it can occur almost anywhere in the cerebral hemispheres and can produce a large variety of neurological syndromes. Recently, the diagnosis of intracerebral hemorrhage has been made much more accurate and easy by the introduction of computerized axial tomography (CAT scan) which readily shows hemorrhages of one centimeter or larger. It is interesting that many clinical situations which were previously thought to be due to cerebral infarction have now been found to be due to small intracerebral hemorrhages. These can be found in any portion of the cerebral hemispheres. Primary intracerebral hemorrhage associated with hypertension is a very serious disorder, carrying an enormously high mortality. Mortality is nearly 95 percent in patients who are rendered comatose, and almost 50 percent in those patients who have serious neurological disability.

There are usually no prior warnings of primary intracerebral hemorrhage. The only clear connection is that with hypertension, and it is one of the major and most serious complications of longstanding hypertension. Patients who have been treated effectively for hypertension have a much lower incidence of primary intracerebral hemorrhage than those who are not treated. Clearly, the treatment of hypertension is the only effective means of preventing primary intracerebral hemorrhage.[13,37] Once primary intracerebral hemorrhage has occurred and the patient has a neurological deficit, the only effective medical therapy is to care for the patient during the life-threatening period of this illness and hope that some spontaneous recovery will occur. Frequently, patients with small hemorrhages will recover with very little, if any, deficit. In general, however, the tendency is for patients to have major deficits and major residuals if they survive the episode. Even in those patients with serious neurological disability where the chances of surviving are slight, hypertension, when present, should be immediately reduced by either the use of intramuscular reserpine, intravenous alpha methyldopa, or rarely, sodium nitroprusside. Blood pressure should be maintained at normal levels or as near normal as possible.

Surgical removal of primary intracerebral hemorrhage has been attempted frequently over the years by neurosurgeons with no evidence that it affects the outcome of the illness or reduces neurological disability. It is possible that with the introduction of computerized axial tomography more definitive analysis of this particular problem may be possible. For those patients who survive primary intracerebral hemorrhages recurrence is uncommon, but they should receive an antihypertensive medication for the remainder of their lives or at least as long as blood pressure remains abnormally elevated.

Ruptured arteriovenous anomaly with intracerebral hemorrhage and subarachnoid hemorrhage is an uncommon event, and one which has symptoms similar to those of primary subarachnoid hemorrhage. The pathophysiology of the condition is related to the rupture of a collection of abnormal cerebral vessels. These collections can vary from being microscopic in size to grossly distorted vascular channels occupying an entire cerebral hemisphere. The vessels in an arteriovenous anomaly are usually abnormal, thin walled structures which are prone to rupture and bleed. Small bleeds frequently occur around the arteriovenous anomaly, damaging brain tissue, and large bleeds may occur, causing major neurological deficit. When the bleeding occurs near the surface of the brain, subarachnoid hemorrhage accompanies the intracerebral hemorrhage. Immediate treatment of the primary event is not different from that of subarachnoid hemorrhage from ruptured aneurysm or from primary intracerebral hemorrhage. There is, however, a high incidence of seizure disorders in patients who suffer from arteriovenous anomalies and the seizures must be treated as outlined in Chapter X of this volume. Surgical removal should be considered after angiographic demonstration of the extent of the anomaly and its arterial supply. Blocking of the many abnormal arterial channels with artificial emboli made of plastic or metal spheres has been attempted with some evidence of benefit.

HYPERTENSIVE ENCEPHALOPATHY

Hypertensive encephalopathy is an acute neurological emergency associated with markedly elevated blood pressure.[43] It occurs only in patients with hypertension and in those, for reasons that are not clear, who have a sudden marked elevation in blood pressure. The pathophysiology of the condition has always been believed to be abnormal vasoconstriction in the face of increased blood pressure, which is marked enough to produce cerebral ischemia and edema around vessels, this occurring in multiple sites. Recently, however, the possibility has been raised that hypertensive encephalopathy is actually related to a "blow-out" phenomenon, in that the vessel is unable any longer to sustain contraction against the increased intraluminal blood pressure. It becomes dilated with a change in its permeability, with seepage of fluid around the vessel and some ischemia. Hypertensive encephalopathy tends to be a generalized brain disorder with spotty areas of ischemia and edema. It more commonly produces changes in personality and states of awareness than it does gross neurological defects. Seizures and visual disturbances are common. Once the diagnosis is made, the most effective treatment is to rapidly reduce the blood pressure. If this cannot be done by intramuscular reserpine or alpha-methyldopa, a sodium nitroprusside drip should be utilized and continued until blood pressure is maintained at normal or near normal levels. Sodium nitroprusside should be given by intravenous infusion in a concentration of .1mg/ml at a rate of about 4–5 drops per minute. Using this method, blood pressure can be brought to any desired level. Treatment of hypertension by this method requires constant supervision to avoid serious hypotension. Diazoxide given intravenously in doses of 300 mg will usually promptly lower blood pressure. Usually the condition is rapidly reversed by lowering the blood pressure and bringing hypertension under control. If blood pressure is not rapidly reduced and hypertension controlled, the disorder carries a high level of mortality.[43]

TEMPORAL ARTERITIS

Temporal arteritis is a serious inflammatory disease of the temporal artery and its branches, and often involves other arteries around the head.[29,11,34] It is usually a disease of elderly people and should be suspected when an elderly person first starts having unilateral headaches. Generally it is associated with inflammation, edema and swelling around the temporal artery which becomes quite tender and sore when pressed. It is often enough associated with loss of vision that it can be an extremely serious disorder. It is almost invariably associated with an elevated sedimentation rate and when treated with corticosteroids, it is promptly relieved. Treatment with steroids should consist initially of 40 mg prednisone daily. Patients are then maintained on this treatment in declining doses with maintenance doses of 5 to 10 mg prednisone per day for several months.[29,11,34]

REFERENCES

1. ADAMS RD, TORVIK A, FISHER CM: Progressing stroke pathogenesis. 3rd Conference on Cerebrovascular Disease. ed. Millikan, C. H., Siekert RG, and Whisnant JP p. 133 New York Grune and Stratton, 1961.
2. BARNETT HJM: The Canadian cooperative stroke study group. A randomized trial of aspirin and sulfinpyrazone in threatened stroke. N. Engl. J. Med. 299: 53, 1978.
3. CARTER AB: Anticoagulant therapy. 3rd Conference on Cerebrovascular Disease. (eds.) Millikan C. H., Siekert, R. G. and Whisnant, J. P. p 151 New York Grune & Stratton, 1961.
4. CARTER AB: The immediate treatment of cerebral embolism. Quart J Med 26: 335, 1957.
5. CARTER AB: Prognosis of cerebral embolism. Lancet 2:514, 1965.
6. DE WIESE JA, ROB CG, SATRAN R et al: Results in carotid endarterectomy for transient ischemic attacks—5 years later. Ann Surg 178:258, 1973.
7. EASTON JD, SHERMAN DG: Stroke and mortality rate in carotid endarterectomy, 228 consecutive operations. Stroke 8: 565, 1977.
8. EVANS G: Effect of platelet-suppressive agents on the incidence of amaurosis fugax and transient cerebral ischemia. McDowell FH and Brennan, RW (eds) Cerebral Vascular Diseases Eighth Conference New York. Grune and Stratton, p 297, 1973.
9. FIELDS WS, LEMATI NA, FRANKOWSKI RF, HARDY RJ: Controlled trial of aspirin in cerebral ischemia. Stroke 8: 301, 1977.
10. FIELDS WS, MASLENIKOV V, MEYER JS et al: Joint study of extracranial arterial occlusion. Progress report of prognosis following surgical or nonsurgical treatment for transient cerebral ischemic attacks and cervical carotid artery lesions. JAMA 211:1993, 1970.
11. FISHER CM: Ocular palsy in temporal arteritis. Minn Med 42: 1258, 1959.
12. FISHER CM: Use of anticoagulants in cerebral thrombosis. Neurology 8: 311, 1958.
13. FREIS EO: Effect of treatment of hypertension on the occurrence of stroke. 9th Conference on Cerebrovascular Disease (eds) Whisnant JP and Sandok BA p 133 Grune and Stratton New York, 1975.
14. GENTON D, BARNETT HJM, FIELDS WF, GERT M, HOAK JC: Report of Joint Committee for Stroke Resources XIV. Cerebral ischemia role of thrombosis and antithrombotic therapy. Stroke 8: 147, 1977.

15. KATZMAN R, CLASSEN R, KLATZO, I, MEYER JS, PAPPIUS HM, WALTZ, AG: Brain edema in stroke. Report of Joint Committee for Stroke Resources Stroke 8: 509, 1977.

16. KATZMAN R, CLASSEN R, KLATZO I, MEYER JS, PAPPIUS HM WALTZ AG: Brain, edema and stroke. Report of Joint Sub Committee for stroke resources. Stroke 8: 512, 1977.

17. McDEVITT E: Anticoagulant therapy in cerebrovascular disease in 3rd conference on cerebrovascular disease. ed. Millikan, CH. New York Grune and Stratton, 1961.

18. McDOWELL FH: Cerebral embolism in Handbook of Clinical Neurology. (eds) Vinken PJ and Bruyn GW 11: North Holland Publishing Co, 1972.

19. McGILL HC, GEER JC, STRONG JP: Natural history of human atherosclerotic lesions in atherosclerosis and its origin. (ed) Sandler M, Bournes GH Academic Press New York 1963.

20. MILLIKAN CH: Reassessment of anticoagulant therapy in various types of occlusive cerebrovascular disease. Stroke 2: 201, 1971.

21. MILLIKAN CH: Reassessment of anticoagulant therapy in various types of occlusive cerebrovascular disease. Stroke 2: 205, 1971.

22. MILLIKAN CH, McDOWELL FH: Treatment of transient ischemic attacks. Stroke 9:299, 1978.

23. MULLAN S, DAWLEY J: Antifibrinolytic therapy for intracranial aneurysms. J Neurosurg 28: 21, 1968.

24. MUNDALL J, QUINTERO P, VONKAULLA KN, HARMON R, AUSTIN J: Transient monocular blindness and increased platelet aggregability treated with aspirin, a case report. Neurology 22: 280, 1972.

25. NIBBELINK DW: Cooperative aneurysm study, antifibrinolytic therapy following subarachnoid hemorrhage from ruptured intracranial aneurysm. 9th Conference on Cerebrovascular Disease (eds) Whisnant JP Sandok BA p. 155 Grune and Stratton New York, 1975.

26. NIBBELINK DW, TORNER JC, HENDERSON WG: Intracranial aneurysm and sub-arachnoid hemorrhage. A cooperative study. Antifibrinolytic therapy recent onset subarachnoid hemorrhage. Stroke 6: 622, 1975.

27. OLSSON JD, MULLER R, BERNEK S: Long term anticoagulation therapy for TIA and minor strokes with minimum residuum. Stroke 7: 444, 1976.

28. PATTERSON RH, HARPEL P: The effect of epsilon-amino caproic acid and tranexamic acid on thrombus size and strength in a simulated arterial aneurysm. J Neurosurg 34:365, 1971.

29. RUSSELL RWR: Giant cell arteritis. Quart J Med 28: 471, 1959.

30. SAHS AL, PERRET GE, LOCKSLEY HB, et al: Intracranial aneurysms and subarachnoid hemorrhage - A cooperative study. Philadelphia JB Lippincott Co., 1969.

31. SANTOS-BUCH CA, GOODHUE WW, EWALD BH: Experimental production of miliary aneurysms with hypertension. 9th Conference on Cerebrovascular Disease (eds) Whisnant JP Sandok BA p. 91 Grune & Stratton, New York.

32. SCHEINBERG P, MEYER JS, REIVICH M, SUNDT TM, WALTZ AG: Cerebral circulation and metabolism in stroke. Report of Joint Committee for Stroke Resources. Stroke 7: 213, 1976.

33. SIEKERT RG, WHISNANT JP, MILLIKAN CH: Surgical and anticoagulant therapy of occlusive cerebral vascular disease. Ann. Intern. Med. 58: 637, 1963.

34. SORENSEN PS, LORENZEN I: Giant cell arteritis, temporal arteritis, and polymyalgia rheumatica. A retrospective study of 63 patients. Acta Med Scand 201: 207, 1977.
35. THOMPSON JE: Surgery for cerebrovascular insufficiency (stroke) Springfield, Ill. Chas C Thomas, 1968.
36. TOOLE JF, PATEL AN: Cerebrovascular Disorders New York Blakiston, 1967.
37. VETERANS ADMINISTRATION COOPERATIVE STUDY GROUP on antihypertensive agents. Effects of treatment on morbidity in hypertension I. Results in patients with diastolic blood pressures averaging 115 through 129 mmHg JAMA 202:1028, 1967.
38. WELLS CE: Cerebral embolism, the natural history, prognostic signs and effects of anticoagulants. Arch Neurol Psychiat 81: 667, 1959.
39. WELLS CE, URREA O: Cerebrovascular accidents in patients receiving anticoagulant drugs. Arch Neurol 3:553, 1960.
40. WHISNANT JP: Discussion. 3rd Conference on Cerebrovascular Disease. (eds.) Millikan, C. H., Siekert, R. G., and Whisnant JP p. 156 Grune and Stratton, New York.
41. WHISNANT JP, ELVEBACK LR, MATSUMOTO N: Effect of duration of treatment with anticoagulants on the prognosis of transient cerebral ischemic attacks. Ninth conference on Cerebrovascular Disease. (eds) Whisnant JP, Sandok BA Grune and Stratton. New York 1975, 187.
42. WRIGHT IS, McDEVITT E, Cerebral vascular diseases, their significance, diagnosis and present treatment, including the selective use of anticoagulant substances. Lancet 2: 825, 1954.
43. ZIEGLER D: Hypertensive vascular disease of the brain. eds. Vinken PJ, Bruyn GW Handbook of Clinical Neurology 11: 552 North Holland Publishing Co New York, 1972.

FURTHER READING

SCHEINBERG, PERITZ (eds): Tenth Princeton Conference, Cerebrovascular Diseases, Raven Press New York, 1976.
WHISNANT JP SANDOK BA (eds): Ninth Princeton Conference, Cerebrovascular Diseases Grune and Stratton, New York, 1975.
McDOWELL, FH and BRENNAN, RW (eds): Eighth Princeton Conference, Cerebrovascular Diseases Grune and Stratton, New York, 1973.
WOLFF, HG: Headache and Other Head Pain, Dalessio, DJ (ed): Oxford Univ Press, 1972.
NELSON, ER (ed) Eleventh Princeton Conferences, Cerebrovascular Diseases Raven Press, New York, 1980.
SCHEINBERG P MEYER JS REIVICH M et al Cerebral Circulation and Metabolism in Stroke, Stroke 7:213–234, 1976.
MARSHALL, JOHN: The Management of Cerebrovascular Disease Blackwell Scientific Publications London, 1976.
TOOLE, JF and PATEL AN: Cerebrovascular Disorders 2nd Ed McGraw-Hill New York, 1974.

SAHS, AL, and HARTMAN EC (eds): Fundamentals of Stroke Care, DHEW Publication, 1976.

CARTER, BARHAM: Cerebral Infarction The MacMillan Co New York, 1964.

SAHS AL, PERRET GE, LOCKSLEY HB, et al Intracranial Aneurysms and Subarachnoid Hemorrhage JB Lippincott Company, Philadelphia, 1969.

5

Myasthenia Gravis (M.G.)

Myasthenia gravis is clinically characterized by weakness of the muscles. This weakness has the tendency to increase upon repeated activity and as the day progresses. Most frequently involved are those muscles that execute the extraocular movements resulting in diplopia, but other bulbar as well as skeletal muscles may often be involved. If the extremities are involved, the weakness is more relatively marked in the distal, as compared to the proximal muscles. The age of onset varies, women are more often afflicted than men. Babies born to myasthenic mothers may show transient myasthenia and require temporary treatment.[11,14,22]

The incidence of myasthenia gravis in the general population is 0.01 to 0.05 percent. Familial incidence, however, is 3 to 5 percent, suggesting a hereditary disposition to susceptibility to myasthenia gravis.[11]

Abnormalities of thymus are frequent among patients suffering from myasthenia gravis, and surgical removal of thymus has often alleviated the myasthenic symptoms.[3,16] The crises in myasthenia are cholinergic, usually resulting from overdosing with anticholinesterase; and myasthenic, resulting from an increased need for acetylcholine and are medical emergencies.[14]

PATHOPHYSIOLOGY

The basic defect in myasthenia gravis appears to be impaired neuromuscular transmission.[11,22] The exact mechanism of this defect is not yet entirely clear. All the evidence accumulated through various pharmacological, biochemical, immunological and electrophysiological studies point to the myoneural junction as the site of the defect. Over the years, theories considering all logical possibilities regarding the nature of the defect at the junction have been offered.[22] Investigators looking for a presynaptic defect have postulated a disturbance in the transmitter i.e., the acetylcholine (AcCh) production, release or recycling. Other investigators looking for a postsynaptic defect, have postulated decreased responsiveness to the transmitter at the endplate. Still others have considered the existence of circulating inhibitor substance(s) that may act either pre- or postsynaptically.

Currently accepted by the majority of investigators as a key finding, is the reduction of the miniature endplate potentials at the myasthenic myoneural junction.[8] The initial interpretation of this phenomenon was that the quanta of AcCh from the presynaptic terminal vesicles were smaller than normal.[8] There is a growing body of evidence, however, that the postsynaptic acetylcholine receptor substance (AcChR) is defective in the myasthenic endplate. Autoradiographic studies using as a marker labeled α-bungarotoxin, which binds irreversibly with AcChR, have shown marked diminution of AcChR in the myasthenic endplates.[11,15] Electronmicroscopic studies have demonstrated a reduction and degenerative changes of the foldings of the myasthenic endplate.[11] Furthermore, circulating antibodies contained in the immunoglobulin G fractions, which react with the AcChR, have been found in the serum of the majority of myasthenic patients thus studied.[15,17] Immunizing experimental animals with purified AcChR causes progressive weakness and diminished miniature endplate potentials, while the titers of antibodies are elevated. It appears then that a major factor in the genesis of myasthenia gravis is damage to AcChR and/or reduction of the amount of AcChR substance caused by the circulating antibodies against AcChR, an autoimmune mechanism. The antibodies against AcChR are thought to be produced in thymus. However, what mechanism sets off the production of antibodies against AcChR remains to be elucidated.[24]

THERAPY

Generally, two therapeutic approaches are being used to overcome the block of neuromuscular transmission, caused presumably by autoimmune mechanisms in myasthenia gravis. The first approach is to administer agents with anticholinesterase action which increase and/or prolong the activity of the transmitter acetylcholine. The second approach is to suppress the autoimmune response by administering steroids, or by thymectomy. Both approaches may be used in combination. The first approach is usually used in milder cases, the second or the combination, in more severe forms.[11,22]

Anticholinesterase Therapy

The agents displaying anticholinesterase effects act by competing for the enzyme with acetylcholine at the cholinergic synapses. They are hydrolyzed by acetylcholine esterase at a lower rate than acetylcholine, therefore sufficient concentration of the drug must be present for effective competition. Agents that do not significantly enter into the central nervous system are preferable, thus minimizing the central side effects.

Historically, physostigmine was the first agent of this category used for the treatment of myasthenia gravis. Central side effects, however, are prominent with physostigmine, because it easily penetrates the blood-brain barriers.

Currently used anticholinesterases include neostigmine, pyridostigmine and ambenonium.[11,14,22] Edrophonium serves as a diagnostic aid.[20] Atropine is often used to alleviate the systemic peripheral muscarinic side effects of anticholinesterases, such as intestinal cramps, salivation, bronchospasm, and diarrhea. Atropine has little effect on nicotinic receptors i.e., it does not counteract the anticholinesterases at myoneural junctions.[14] Long-acting anticholinesterases such as organo-phosphates have not been successful in the treatment of myasthenia gravis.[1]

Neostigmine has a relatively short half-life as it is rapidly inactivated. The inactivation starts in the intestinal tract, which explains the marked differences in the size of the effective parenteral and oral doses. The short half-life also necessitates frequent administration of doses, every 2 to 6 hours in maintenance therapy.[14]

The starting oral dose is usually 15 mg administered three times daily. Starting with low dosages alleviates the intensity of its muscarinic side effects. The dose is then built up according to the individual patient's need, reaching on the average 120 to 180 mg daily, taken in 15 or 30 mg installments every 2 to 6 hours, with an average of 4 hour intervals.

Parenterally, 0.5 to 1.0 mg is usually equivalent to 15 mg taken orally, subject to individual variations. The parenteral route is used mostly in treating the myasthenic crises, which will be discussed separately.

The common muscarinic side effects of neostigmine are nausea, vomiting, diarrhea, and intestinal cramps; increased perspiration, salivation, lacrimation, and bronchial secretion; less often hypotension. With gross overdose, cholinergic crisis will ensue and enough neostigmine may enter the central nervous system to cause agitation, mental clouding and coma.

The side effects associated with the common doses of neostigmine are alleviated by oral administration of 0.3 to 0.6 mg of atropine sulfate 2 to 6 times daily.[14]

Pyridostigmine is longer acting than neostigmine, thus doses need to be given every 3 to 8 hours.[11,14,22] The oral dose of pyridostigmine equivalent to 15 mg of neostigmine is 60 mg. Plasma levels of 20 to 60 ng/ml have been observed in patients receiving effective doses of pyridostigmine.[4,5] Parenterally 1.0 mg of pyridostigmine has usually the same effects as 0.5 mg of neostigmine. The side effects of the two drugs are similar.

Ambenonium is effective longer than pyridostigmine or neostigmine, and allows longer intervals between doses. The oral dose equivalent to 15 mg of neostigmine is 5 mg of ambenonium. The side effects are similar to those of other anticholinesterases but ambenonium appears to penetrate the blood-brain barrier to a somewhat greater extent than neostigmine and pyridostigmine. Therefore, central side effects may limit the use of high doses of ambenonium.[11,14,22]

Edrophonium, due to its very brief action, is impractical for maintenance therapy but is useful primarily as a diagnostic agent. Given intravenously in a dose of 10 mg, it markedly reduces the myasthenic weakness within seconds, for a few minutes. Non-myasthenic weak muscles may also respond, but the effect is briefer and much less dramatic than in myasthenic muscles. Cholinergic crises can be differentiated from myasthenic crises (in an intensive care unit) by injecting 2 or 5 mg of edrophonium. The patient in myasthenic crisis improves dramatically; the patient in cholinergic crisis either does not change or becomes worse for a short period.[11,20]

Although the anticholinesterase therapy is quite effective in many patients, it rarely reconstitutes full function of all muscles. It alleviates the symptoms enough, however, to allow a reasonably normal life. There is some experimental evidence that prolonged high dose anticholinesterase treatment leads to morphologic and degenerative changes at the myoneural junction. It has been postulated that the same may contribute to the degenerative changes seen in some long-term myasthenic patients. Therefore immunosuppressive therapy is used more often now than in earlier years, particularly if the response to reasonable doses of anticholinesterases is less than satisfactory.

Immunosuppressive Chemotherapy

The use of immunosuppressive agents such as prednisone and corticotrophin has become an important supplement to the anticholinesterase therapy in selected myasthenic patients.[10,11] The initial worsening of myasthenic symptoms from immunosuppressive agents can be minimized by appropriate dosing schedules and by the preparedness to cope with transient worsenings. A marked long-term improvement of myasthenia often follows, allowing substantial reductions from the previous anticholinesterase requirements.

The selection of immunosuppressive agents and the administration schedules are still in flux and are likely to be modified as the general experience grows. It should be noted that the majority, but not all patients, have responded favorably to this form of treatment.

The patients selected for treatment with immunosuppressive agents usually are those with generalized myasthenia, who do not respond well to the average doses of anticholinesterases. Among the patients who benefitted from immunosuppression, many have had thymectomy, others responded favorably only after they were thymectomized. Patients with only ocular myasthenia are included if disabled by distortions of vision. Excluded are usually patients to whom the common side effects of steroid treatment (gastrointestinal bleeding, electrolyte disturbances, impaired resistance to infection etc.) are likely to pose undue risks. These include patients with peptic ulcers, diabetes mellitus and cardiovascular diseases.[2,10,18]

The initiation of steroid treatment is best carried out in facilities where the potential initial worsening of myasthenic symptoms can be quickly and expertly coped with, such as intensive care units or neurology inpatient wards. The common steroid side effects are minimized by reducing sodium and supplementing potassium intake as well as by administration of antacids.

Corticotrophin   Historically, corticotrophin was the first immunoactive agent used.[21] On the average, 100 units can be infused intravenously over an 8 hour period or 160 units given intramuscularly for 8 to 14 days. More than one course at intervals of 7 to 10 days may be given, if no improvement occurs or only transient effect is seen. The maintenance doses of 100 units weekly are then continued for months, as indicated.[2] This form of treatment is currently generally used when all other forms of therapy have failed. The incidence of initial worsening of myasthenia is highest with this agent, therefore the early phases of corticotrophin therapy are carried out in intensive care units. Antacids and potassium supplements are given as needed.[2,10,11]

Prednisone,   a synthetic glucocorticoid which has a short plasma half-life, undergoes biotransformation and is eliminated in the urine. It is well absorbed following oral ingestion. The dosages of prednisone used successfully have ranged from 50 to 100 mg given as a single oral dose every other day. The alternate day schedule seems to reduce the adrenal-pituitary suppression.[25] Starting with a low, such as a 25 mg dose, followed by increases might minimize the occurrence of the initial worsening of myasthenic symptoms.[23] Improvement on this high alternate day dosage schedule is usually seen in a couple of months. Later the maintenance dose can be reduced very gradually

(2.5 to 5.0 mg per month) to near one half or less from the earlier maximum, depending upon the individual patient's response. In some patients prednisone can be discontinued eventually.[2,10,18,25]

The anticholinesterase drugs may be withdrawn at the onset of prednisone therapy but more often it may be practical to continue them. The amount of anticholinesterase needed, however, diminishes considerably, if the prednisone becomes effective.[10]

It is advisable to monitor and regulate sodium and potassium balance during prednisone therapy as well as to administer antacids, as needed.

Thymectomy

The long-term empirical experience has demonstrated that thymectomy has been beneficial in a good number of myasthenic patients.[3,12] It may be viewed as another immunosuppressive measure. The most dramatic improvement of myasthenia from the thymectomy has been observed in young adult women. With present day technology, the surgical risk is generally small. Postoperatively, the anticholinesterases are administered parenterally until regular oral intake becomes possible.[3,12,16,18]

Plasmapheresis

Another way to remove circulating immunoactive material from the organism is plasmapheresis. This has been used experimentally and has resulted in improvement of myasthenic symptoms for variable periods.[6] The complicity and cost of this procedure, however, limit its general clinical application at present time.

Myasthenia of Newborns

Babies born to mothers with myasthenia gravis may show myasthenic symptoms and need anticholinesterase therapy in order to survive.[13] This is probably a reaction to passively transferred immunoactive agents from the mother that affect AcCh receptors in the newborn. Repeated 0.1 mg intramuscular doses of neostigmine may be needed in the first days of life. The condition usually improves in the following days and abates in a week or two.

Crises in Myasthenic Patients

Sometimes a rapid increase of muscle weakness to the extreme, including respiratory muscles, occurs in patients with myasthenia gravis. Two mechanisms are recognized: (1) myasthenic crises and (2) cholinergic crises.

The myasthenic crises occur when the patient ran out of medicine or there is an increased need of anticholinesterase drug. Cholinergic crises are caused by an excess of AcCh at the myoneural junction, usually from excessive intake of anticholinesterases. Both are medical emergencies.[11,14,22]

Until edrophonium became available the two forms of crises were differentiated by withholding medication while supporting respiration as needed. The patient in myasthenic crisis remains weak, while the patient in cholinergic crisis improves upon withholding medication.

Edrophonium 2 or 5 mg given intravenously will establish within minutes the diagnosis between myasthenic and cholinergic crises. Rapid transient improvement occurs in the patient with myasthenic crisis, while the patient in cholinergic crisis becomes worse.[20] The most significant indicator for the edrophonium effect in this setting is a change in the respiratory function and volume.

Treatment of Myasthenic Crises

Factors that may lead to myasthenic crises other than inadvertent stopping of medication include intercurrent infection, trauma, either accidental or surgical, several drugs such as neomycin, quinine, quinidine and, of course, curare-like agents.

The treatment is carried out in an intensive care unit and consists of maintaining adequate respiratory ventilation and giving anticholinesterase parenterally. Neostigmine (0.5 mg) intramuscularly or subcutaneously is given every 15 to 30 minutes until desired response is seen. After the required dose to maintain adequate function has been established, pyridostigmine may be substituted as it has a longer action. Later, when the patient has completely stabilized, oral medication can be resumed. Atropine is given as needed to counteract the side effects.

Treatment of Cholinergic Crises

The cholinergic crises are best treated by stopping medication and waiting, to allow excess medication to be hydrolyzed *in situ*. It would seem that logical chemotherapeutic agents in this situation would be antidotes used for treatment of excessive exposure to insecticides containing organophosphorus. However, these agents are rarely needed. Supportive measures are applied as needed, primarily to maintain adequate pulmonary ventilation. Atropine may be administered to alleviate the muscarinic side effects.

Pseudomyasthenia (Lambert-Eaton Syndrome)

A myasthenic syndrome characterized by weakness in mostly proximal extremity muscle groups is to be differentiated from myasthenia gravis.[7,9] It improves only slightly with anticholinesterases and shows diagnostic electromyographic patterns. The incidence of lung cancer among patients thus afflicted is high.

Lambert-Eaton syndrome or pseudomyasthenia responds well to guanidine, which is thought to act by increasing the number of quanta of acetylcholine released from the nerve terminals.[19] The maintenance dosages range from 1.0 to 2.5 gm daily but it is advisable to start with 250 mg of guanidine twice or three times daily. Diarrhea and intestinal cramps occur as side effects; skin rashes have been observed in some patients.

REFERENCES

1. ARANOW H JR, HOEFER PFA, ROWLAND LP: Long-acting anticholinesterase drugs in the management of myasthenia gravis. J Chronic Dis 6: 457, 1957.
2. BRUNNER NG, BERGER CL, NAMBA T, GROB D: Corticotrophin and corticosteroids in generalized myasthenia gravis: Comparative studies and role in management. Ann NY Acad Sci 274: 577–595, 1976.
3. BUCKINGHAM JM, HOWARD FM JR, BERNATZ PE et al: The value of thymectomy in myasthenia gravis: A computer-assisted matched study. Ann Surg 184: 453–458, 1976.
4. CALVEY TN, CHAN K: Plasma pyridostigmine levels in patients with myasthenia gravis. Clin Pharmacol Ther 21: 187–193, 1977.
5. COHAN SL, DRETCHEN KL, NEAL A: Malabsorption of pyridostigmine in patients with myasthenia gravis. Neurology 27: 299–301, 1977.
6. DAU PC, LINDSTROM JM, CASSELL CK, et al: Plasmapheresis and immunosuppressive drug therapy in myasthenia gravis. N Engl J Med 297: 1134–1140, 1977.
7. EATON LM, LAMBERT EH: Electromyography and electrical stimulation of nerves in diseases of motor unit: Observations on myasthenic syndrome associated with malignant tumors. JAMA 163: 1117–1124, 1957.
8. ELMQVIST D, HOFMANN WW, KUGELBERG J, et al: An electrophysiological investigation on neuromuscular transmission in myasthenia gravis. J Physiol (London) 174: 417–437, 1964.
9. ELMQVIST D, LAMBERT E: Neuromuscular transmission in the patient with myasthenic syndrome sometimes associated with bronchogenic carcinoma. Mayo Clinic Proc 43: 689–694, 1968.
10. ENGEL WK: Myasthenia, corticosteroids, anticholinesterases. Ann NY Acad Sci 274: 623–630, 1976.
11. ENGEL WK, FESTOFF BW, PATTEN BM, et al: Myasthenia gravis. Ann Int Med 81: 225–246, 1974.

12. FAULKNER SL, EHYAI A, FISHER RD et al: Contemporary management of myasthenia gravis. The clinical role of thymectomy. Ann Thorac Surg 23: 248–252, 1977.
13. FENICHEL GM: Clinical syndromes of myasthenia in infancy and childhood. A review. Arch Neurol 35: 97–103, 1978.
14. FLACKE W: Treatment of myasthenia gravis. N Engl J Med 288: 27–35, 1973.
15. KEESEY J, SHAIKH I, WOLFGRAM F, et al: Studies on the ability of acetylcholine receptors to bind alpha-bungarotoxin after exposure to myasthenic serum. Ann NY Acad Sci 274: 244–253, 1976.
16. KEYNES G: The results of thymectomy in myasthenia gravis. Br Med J II: 611–616, 1949.
17. LEFVERT AK, PRISKANEN R: Acetylcholine receptor antibodies in cerebrospinal fluid of patients with myasthenia gravis. Lancet 2: 351–352, 1977.
18. MANN JD, JOHNS TR, CAMPA JF, et al: Long-term prednisone followed by thymectomy in myasthenia gravis. Ann NY Acad Sci 274: 608–622, 1976.
19. OH SJ, KIM KW: Guanidine hydrochloride in the Eaton-Lambert syndrome. Electrophysiological improvement. Neurology 23: 1084–1090, 1973.
20. OSSERMAN KE, GENKINS G: Critical appraisal of the use of edrophonium (Tensilon) chloride tests in myasthenia gravis and significance of clinical classification. Ann NY Acad Sci 135: 312, 1966.
21. VON REIS G, LILJESTRAND A, MATELL G: Treatment of severe myasthenia gravis with large doses of ACTH. Ann NY Acad Sci 135: 409–416, 1966.
22. ROWLAND LP: Myasthenia gravis. In: *Scientific Approaches to Clinical Neurology.* Eds: ES Goldensohn, SH Appel. Lea and Febiger, Philadelphia, 1518–1554, 1977.
23. SEYBOLD ME, DRACHMAN DB: Gradually increasing doses of prednisone in myasthenia gravis. N Engl J Med 290: 81–88, 1974.
24. SIMPSON JA: Myasthenia gravis: A personal view of pathogenesis and mechanism. Muscle and Nerve 1: 151–156, 1978.
25. WARMOLTS JR, ENGEL WK: Benefit from alternate-day prednisone in myasthenia gravis. N Engl J Med 286: 17–20, 1972.

6

Multiple Sclerosis

Multiple sclerosis is clinically characterized by neurological signs originating from disseminated, relatively small focal lesions in the central nervous system. Often involved are vision, extraocular movements, limb movements and sensation, and bladder control. The signs and symptoms may remit completely after the initial episode, but later exacerbate and the clinical picture may then involve new symptoms. As the disease progresses, remissions tend to become incomplete and the exacerbation more severe, leading to episodically increasing disability over the years.[4,15]

The nature of this disease is unclear. Demyelination is found in the focal areas of the central nervous system with changes of lipid profiles in the involved areas.[15] What sets off the demyelinizing process is unknown. Hypotheses regarding the etiology of multiple sclerosis suggest (1) viral infection, (2) disturbance in immuno-mechanism and (3) abnormalities in lipid metabolism, among others.[1,12,14,15] It has also been thought that part of the dysfunction during an acute exacerbation is caused by the pressure effect on adjacent structures from the focal area.[15]

Specific therapy of multiple sclerosis has been and still is a vexing problem.[16,19,20] Due to the waxing and waning nature of the disease, evaluation of the effectiveness of any form of therapy of multiple sclerosis is extremely difficult. It appears, so far, that a clear-cut beneficial influence on the general course of the disease has not been achieved with any of the attempted treatment regimens. Agents that have been tried and failed to have proven effectiveness are numerous.[19,20] They include isoniazid, tolbutamide, dicumarol, heparin, chloroquine, clofibrate, cyanocobalamin, methotrexate, cytarabine, cyclophosphamide, azathiorine, and antilymphocytic globulin, among many others. Corticotrophin and corticosteroids, though beneficially modify the course of an acute exacerbation, have not clearly modified the general course of the disease in long-term therapy.[17]

In the long-term treatment of multiple sclerosis, supportive measures, adequate diet, and a cautiously optimistic attitude on the part of the managing physician are best for the patient's well-being and morale. Vitamin supplements in moderate doses are not harmful and may have a temporarily positive placebo effect in some patients.

STEROID TREATMENT

If no long-term cure has been found for multiple sclerosis through chemotherapy so far, the course of an acute exacerbation may nevertheless be alleviated with steroid treatment.[3,17] Short courses of high doses of corticotrophin or corticosteroids are used.

Corticotrophin gel may be given intramuscularly for a 2 to 3 week period. A high dose of 80 to 120 units per day may be given in the first week, followed by a gradual reduction of the dose in the final week of the course. Such short courses seldom cause serious complications if the electrolyte balance is monitored and antacids are given as needed. Patients who also have diabetes mellitus, peptic ulcer, hypertension, systemic infections or psychoses must be excluded from this form of treatment.

Prednisone may be used for the treatment of acute exacerbations of multiple sclerosis. It is usually given for a period of 3 to 6 weeks. A high dose, 80 to 100 mg per day, is used initially, followed by a gradual reduction of the dose in the final week of the course. Again, this form of therapy can not be used in patients with contraindications to steroid therapy.

In long-term management of patients with multiple sclerosis the common problems one has to deal with include constipation, genitourinary infections and spasticity.[3,13,15,20] Laxatives are used as needed, fecal impaction is to be avoided. Urinary tract infections are common in patients with long-standing disease, particularly if indwelling catheters are needed because of incontinence.[13] Proper catheter hygiene is important and appropriate antimicrobial agents are used, depending upon the type of organism and its sensitivity.[15,20]

Spasticity, either in the form of stiffness or frequent flexor spasms may become a distressing problem in patients with multiple sclerosis. Several considerations are required in dealing with this problem. The spasticity in a weak limb may serve a splinting function. Removing the splinting may allow an easier collapse of a somewhat weak leg, thus increasing the difficulties in walking or standing. On the other hand, the spasms and stiffness of the spastic limbs may cause extreme discomfort at times. Thus, influencing the spasticity with treatment may worsen some and improve other symptoms.[3] The treatment plan is to be adjusted accordingly. For treatment schedules, see the section on treatment of spasticity.

SPASTICITY

Spasticity usually develops following lesions of the corticospinal tract. It is characterized by increased resistance to passive stretching of limbs and exaggerated deep tendon reflexes; clonus may also be present. The pathophysiology of spasticity is not well understood, but it may be related to alterations of transmitter balance at synapses and changes in the sensitivity of the muscle spindles.[5,7]

The majority of patients presenting with spasticity are those who have suffered a spinal cord injury, have a spinal cord tumor, degenerative spinal cord disease; or have multiple sclerosis.

The treatment of spasticity is often unsatisfactory. Drugs that have been used with some success are diazepam, baclofen and dantrolene.

Diazepam is thought to relieve spasticity due to its suppressive action on interneuronal pathways and polysynaptic spinal reflexes, associated with a dampening effect on muscle spindles. Clinically, the dosage requirements vary considerably among patients.[5,15,20] A reasonable starting dose is 2 mg twice a day. A sedative effect at the onset of therapy is not unusual, but tolerance to diazepam varies considerably among patients. The dose is then increased in 2 to 5 mg increments until beneficial effect is seen, and many patients tolerate 30 or 40 mg daily without side effects. Unfortunately, the effect of diazepam on spasticity is often not long lasting. In these patients it is advisable to stop the medication and "rest" for a few weeks or months. Initiating therapy later may produce another period of relief.

Side effects with diazepam other than sedation rarely pose problems. Dermatologic, renal, hepatic and hematologic complications are extremely infrequent, but habituation may develop. Discontinuation of diazepam in patients who have received high doses should not be abrupt.

Baclofen 4-amino-3-(p-chlorophenyl)-butyric acid is an analogue of gamma-aminobutyric acid. It is thought to act by augmenting recurrent inhibition through an enhancement of Renshaw cell activity and decreasing the polysynaptic flexor reflex transmission.[18] It is well absorbed from the intestinal tract, peak plasma level occurring in about 2 hours following oral ingestion. Biotransformation of baclofen is not extensive, over 75 percent of the dose is excreted unchanged in the urine. The plasma half-life in man is 3 to 4 hours.[10]

Baclofen does not penetrate the blood-brain barrier easily, nevertheless, it reaches an effective concentration in the spinal cord with adequate doses.

The effective dose varies among patients. It is advisable to start with 5 mg three times daily and increase the dose slowly over weeks until beneficial effect is seen. In recent studies of patients with multiple sclerosis, 70 to 80 mg daily in divided doses were adequate in over 75 percent of patients who did benefit from the drug. Side effects of baclofen include nausea and somnolence, less often, headache, constipation, increased weakness, vertigo and insomnia.[8,11,18]

Dantrolene is thought to act by blocking muscle contraction through interference with the calcium mechanism in the muscle cell.[6] The starting dose is 25 mg two or three times daily, increased over 4 to 6 day periods until effective or a maximum of 600 to 800 mg is reached.[9]

The common side effects are diarrhea, nausea and muscle weakness. Less common but more important are potential liver damage, heralded by abnormal liver function tests, which may culminate in a clinical toxic hepatitis.[9] Hallucinations have occurred in some patients receiving dantrolene.[2]

In patients who do not respond to drug therapy and in whom spontaneous improvement is not expected to take place, instillation of phenol intrathecally or surgical rhizotomy may have to be resorted to.

REFERENCES

1. Alter M: Is multiple sclerosis an age-dependent host-response to measles? Lancet 1: 456–457, 1976.
2. Andrews LG, Ashok MS, Pinkerton AC: Hallucinations associated with dantrolene sodium therapy. Can Med Assoc J 112: 148, 1975.
3. Bauer HJ: Problems of symptomatic therapy in multiple sclerosis. Neurology: Vol 28, No 9, Part 2, pp 8–20, 1978.
4. Bauer HJ, Firnhaber W, Winkler W: Prognostic criteria in multiple sclerosis. Ann NY Acad Sci 122: 542, 1965.
5. Burke DJ: An approach to the treatment of spasticity. Drugs 10, 1975.
6. Chyatte SB, Basmajian JV: Dantrolene sodium: Long-term effects in severe spasticity. Arch Phys Med Rehab 54: 311–315, 1973.
7. Davidoff RA: Pharmacology of spasticity. Neurology: Vol 28, No 9, Part 2, pp 46–51, 1978.
8. Duncan GW, Shabani BT, Young RR: An evaluation of baclofen treatment for certain symptoms in patients with spinal cord lesions. Neurology 26: 441–446, 1976.
9. Dykes MH: Evaluation of a muscle relaxant: Datrolene sodium (dantrium). JAMA 231: 862–864, 1975.
10. Faigle JW, Keberle H: The metabolism and pharmacokinetics of Lioresal.

Spasticity: A topical survey. In: An International Symposium, Vienna, 1971. Ed: W Birkmayer, Huber, Vienna, pp 94–100, 1972.
11. FELDMAN RG, KELLY-HAYES M, CONOMY JP, FOLEY JM: Baclofen for spasticity in multiple sclerosis. Neurology 28: 1094–1098, 1978.
12. HAIRE M, FRASER KB, MILLAR JHD: Measles and other virus-specific antibodies in multiple sclerosis. Brit Med J 3: 612, 1973.
13. JAMESON RM: Multiple sclerosis and the urinary tract. Practitioner 218: 91–96, 1977.
14. LAMPERT F, LAMPERT P: Multiple sclerosis: Morphologic evidence of intranuclear paramyxovirus or altered chromatin fibers? Arch Neurol 32: 425–427, 1975.
15. MCALPINE D, LUMSDEN C, ACHESON E: Multiple sclerosis, a reappraisal. Churchill/Livingstone, Edinburgh and London, 1972.
16. MILLER H: The treatment of multiple sclerosis. Practitioner 192: 62, 1964.
17. ROSE AS et al: Cooperative study in the evaluation of therapy in multiple sclerosis: ACTH vs. placebo. Final report. Neurology 20: 1–59, 1970. # 5 Part 2
18. SACHAIS BA, LOGUE IN, CAREY MS: Baclofen, a new antispastic drug. A controlled multicenter trial in patients with multiple sclerosis. Arch Neurol 34: 422–428, 1977.
19. SCHUMACHER GA, BEEBE GW, KIBLER RF et al: Problems of experimental trials of therapy in multiple sclerosis: report by the panel on the evaluation of experimental trials of therapy in multiple sclerosis. Ann NY Acad Sci 122: 552, 1965.
20. SIBLEY WA: Drug treatment of multiple sclerosis. In: Handbook of Clinical Neurology. Vol 9. Eds: PJ Vinken, GW Bruyn. North Holland Publ Co, Amsterdam pp 383, 1970.

7

Head Pain

MIGRAINOUS HEADACHES

Migrainous headaches, also called vascular or essential headaches, include the common and classical migraines and the cluster headaches (migrainous neuralgia or histamine headaches).

It is generally accepted that migraine is associated with cranial vascular changes. During the prodromes, vasoconstriction of the intercranial vessels occurs, leading to various neurological manifestations depending upon the site of major vasoconstriction. During the headache phase, dilatation of extracranial vessels occurs, with edema in the surrounding tissue.[2,11] Migrainous headaches are episodic, with intervals of freedom of headache between attacks. It is not clear what sets off the attacks. A biochemical basis has been postulated that involves alterations in the balance or distribution of monamine transmitters, particularly serotonin, perhaps associated with altered sensitivity of central and peripheral serotonin receptors.[20] This would help to understand why agents that affect serotonin response are effective in the treatment of migraine.

There are two aspects in the management of migrainous patients: (1) amelioration or blocking of an acute attack, and (2) preventive therapy in patients whose attacks are frequent or very severe.

Treatment of Acute Migraine Attack

Mild attacks may respond to salicylates, propoxyphene, or paracetamol. However, if these are unsatisfactory, the drug of first choice is ergotamine tartrate.[7,11,16,24]

Ergotamine tartrate causes vasoconstriction by stimulating alpha-adrenergic receptors and, to some extent, by blocking serotonin receptors.[5,8] In very high doses, however, it may block the alpha-adrenergic receptors. With common clinical doses, its antimigraine effect probably results from vasoconstriction and the reduction of pulsations of the extracranial arteries.[5]

About 60 percent of the dose of ergotamine is absorbed from the intestinal tract.[1] With common clinical doses the peak blood level occurs in 2 hours and is in the low (1–3) nanogram/ml range.[14] Its absorption is facilitated by caffeine. Ergotamine tartrate is most effective if given at the onset of an attack. The usual oral or sublingual dose is 2 mg taken when the pain starts, followed by 2 mg every hour, if necessary, until the pain is relieved, but not exceeding 6 mg per day. Resting in darkness appears to enhance the action of the drug. If a more rapid effect is desirable or if a patient has severe nausea or vomiting with the headaches, a dose of 0.5 mg intramuscularly at the onset of an attack may be given. Other routes of administration of ergotamine are 2 mg rectal suppositories or an aerosol inhaler which delivers 0.36 mg per application. With adequate doses, relief of attacks in 70 percent to 80 percent of the patients can be expected. Ergotamine therapy may be more effective when used together with caffeine, due in part to the improved absorption of ergotamine.[19] Combination preparations containing 1 or 2 mg of ergotamine with 50 or 100 mg of caffeine are available. The advantages of the combined medication, however, may be diminished by insomnia caused by the caffeine; thus its use depends upon an individual patient's preference.

Sometimes a migraine attack continues even after the maximum dose of ergotamine has been taken.[11,16] In those instances, strong analgesics such as codeine or pentazocine may be used. Sedation with barbiturates may be helpful and the inducement of sleep with 100 to 200 mg of pentobarbital has terminated many severe attacks. Flurazepam (15 to 30 mg) can also be used for that purpose. Continuing nausea and vomiting may be treated with antiemetic phenothiazines such as prochlorperazine (5 to 10 mg) or thiethylperazine (6.5 mg) given either as a suppository or parenterally.

Side effects of ergotamine occur in up to 30 percent of treated patients and include numbness and paresthesias of extremities, muscle cramps and stiffness, tiredness, and precordial distress.[11,17,24] They tend to be more frequent and more severe with higher doses. Prolonged overdosage may lead to ergotism, culminating in gangrene of the toes and fingers. Ergotamine tartrate should not be used in patients with severe hypertension or with coronary, cerebral, or peripheral vascular disease, or with impaired kidney or liver function, or sepsis. It is best avoided in pregnancy, but since it has relatively little oxytoxic effect, it may be used with caution, if indicated.

In some patients, ergotamine habituation may become a problem.[11] It is manifested by daily rebound headaches after the effect of ergotamine diminishes a few hours after it has been taken. This vicious circle of continued daily medication can be broken by a supervised "withdrawal" period, during which the headaches are treated with codeine (30 to 45 mg orally) or pentazocine (30 to 45 mg intramuscularly) given at 4 hour intervals, if necessary.

Dihydroergotamine mesylate is also effective in the treatment of acute migraine attacks. Its pharmacological effects are similar to those of ergotamine tartrate, although the vasoconstrictive effect is less and the reflex adrenergic blocking effect is somewhat greater in comparison.[8,15] It is very poorly absorbed from the intestinal tract, therefore it is mostly administered parenterally.[1] The initial dose, given as soon as possible after the signs of an oncoming attack, is 1.0 mg intramuscularly. A similar dose may be given every hour, if needed, until the headache disappears, but not exceeding 3 mg in a day. Intravenous administration of 0.5 mg may be used if a rapid effect is necessary; then the total dose should not exceed 2 mg.

Side effects of dihydroergotamine include those mentioned for ergotamine and the contraindications for the two drugs are the same. Acute overdose of dihydroergotamine has caused hypertension or hypotension, coma, and convulsions. In the treatment of dihydroergotamine overdose, vasodilators may be of some use and diazepam may be given intravenously in case of convulsions.

Preventive Therapy

Therapy for preventing the migraine attacks is indicated in patients who suffer from frequent attacks, i.e., several per week or month. It is also used in patients whose attacks respond little, if at all, to ergotamine treatment or whose attacks are incapacitating. Before embarking on such therapy, aggravating factors should be excluded or treated properly. Among these are arterial hypertension, cervical spondylosis, mental depression or anxiety, oral contraceptives, estrogen therapy, or excessive use of ergotamine. Agents that have been effective in the preventive therapy of migraine are serotonin antagonists such as methysergide, cyproheptadine and pisotifen, and the beta-adrenergic blocker propranolol.[7,11,13,18]

Methysergide is one of the most effective agents in this respect, but has to be used with caution because of potentially severe side effects. Its action is primarily that of a competitive inhibitor of serotonin, antagonizing some effects of serotonin in several organ systems.[5] In large doses it also mimics or enhances the effects of serotonin in maintaining the constriction of scalp arteries.[8] Methysergide is absorbed reasonably well after oral ingestion, the peak plasma level occurring after 1–2 hours.[1] Plasma levels may range between 20–40 ng/ml during the maintenance therapy with common doses.[14] Methysergide reduces the frequency of attacks in approximately 60 percent of patients treated with it, and when the attacks do recur, less ergotamine is usually needed to alleviate an attack.

The dose of methysergide should be increased slowly with a test dose of 0.5 mg given initially to rule out idiosyncracy. If compatible, the dose is then increased over a week from 1 mg daily, to 1 mg three times daily, to 2 mg three times daily. It usually becomes effective in a week or two; if no benefit is seen in a month, there is little reason for continuation of methysergide. If effective, the treatment may be continued for six months, but then withdrawn to forestall development of fibrotic complications.[3,9,21] The withdrawal should be done gradually over 2–3 weeks to avoid rebound headache. The fibrotic complications include retroperitoneal fibrosis, causing backache, girdle feeling, and abdominal pain; pleuropulmonary fibrosis, causing chest pain and dyspnea; or cardiac valvular fibrosis, causing heart murmurs, cardiomegaly, and dyspnea.[9,21] After a drug-free interval of 1–2 months, the drug may be given again for another six months.

During methysergide therapy, nausea, epigastric discomfort, paresthesias, and muscle cramps are relatively common in up to 45 percent of patients treated.[11,21] They are most often seen at the onset of therapy and tend to diminish or disappear during continued therapy or after reduction of the dose. Yet about 10 percent of patients are unable to continue methysergide because of side effects. Close supervision in all patients is mandatory. Methysergide should not be used in patients with active peptic ulcer, severe hypertension, ischemic heart or peripheral vascular disease, thrombophlebitis, renal disease, or pregnancy.

Cyproheptadine, a serotonin antagonist,[13] may be used starting with 2 mg three times daily and building up to 4 mg given three or four times daily, if needed. Sedation frequently occurs at the onset of therapy because of the antihistaminic effect of cyproheptadine. Weight gain occurs in some patients but fibrotic complications have not been observed.

Pisotifen, another serotonin antagonist,[12,13] has been effective in doses up to 3 mg total per day in some patients. It is again advisable to start with a low dose of 0.5 mg three times daily to alleviate its sedative effects. Fibrotic complications have not been reported.

Propranolol has shown promise in the preventive treatment of migraine.[4,6,25] It is considered by some to be almost as effective as methysergide, but potentially less toxic. Propranolol is primarily a blocker of beta-adrenergic receptors. It may prevent migraine attacks by creating a vasoconstrictive bias and preventing the dilatation of extracranial arteries. It may have some effect upon serotonin mechanisms since it has been shown to block serotonin uptake by platelets. Propranolol is adequately absorbed after oral intake, the peak plasma level occurring in 1–2 hours following ingestion.[23]

The effective doses of propranolol in preventing migraine attacks have ranged from 80–240 mg daily with an average 160 mg. The therapy may be started with 20 mg twice a day and the dose built up as needed.[4,6]

Common side effects of propranolol include nausea, abdominal cramps, and diarrhea, postural hypotension, and drowsiness. Fibrotic complications analogous to those of methysergide have not been observed. The dosage should be kept below that level which would lower the heart rate to less than 60 per minute. Propranolol should not be used in patients with asthma, chronic obstructive lung disease, heart disease including congestive failure and atrioventricular conduction disturbances, and diabetes mellitus.

Barbiturates, phenothiazines, and benzodiazepines may be beneficial in migraine prophylaxis by reducing anxiety and modifying reactions to frustration. Tricyclic antidepressants are more efficient than antianxiety agents in some patients, since depression frequently accompanies hard-to-control migraine. Oral contraceptives may reduce the incidence of migraine attacks in some patients, but in others they have provoked or caused the headache de novo; therefore, they should be used with caution and according to an individual patient's response.

Treatment of Cluster Headaches (Migraine Neuralgia)

Cluster headaches are characterized by attacks of severe pain, usually retroorbital, associated with lacrymation and blockage of the nostril on the same side. These attacks occur many times on successive days or weeks, each episode lasting from less than an hour to several hours. There may be free intervals of several months or years between bouts. The drug of choice is methysergide, given in doses of 2 mg three times daily at the onset of the headache, with additional doses up to 12 mg daily, if needed. The dose-related side effects of methysergide (see section on prevention of migraine) occur frequently with these relatively high doses. However, since the clusters usually are limited to a few weeks, the fibrotic complications resulting from long-term administration of high doses are not expected. Parenteral ergotamine tartrate (0.25 mg, 3 to 6 times daily) which was used before the introduction of methysergide, may be used in cases refractory to methysergide.[11,22]

FACIAL PAIN

Three clinical categories of facial pain can be distinguished: (1) typical neuralgias, (2) postherpetic neuralgia, and (3) atypical facial pain.

Typical Neuralgias

Typical neuralgias are manifested by pain in the distribution of the fifth, ninth, and rarely in the tenth cranial nerves.

Trigeminal Neuralgia

Trigeminal neuralgia is characterized by sudden brief bouts of excruciating pain in the sensory distribution of the branches of trigeminal nerve. Most frequently involved is the maxillary branch, but involvement of various combinations of the all three branches occurs as well. The pain is often elicited by tactile stimuli of trigger zones, or by temperature changes such as cold wind or drinking of hot or cold liquids. The onset of the disorder usually occurs in maturity, and women are more often afflicted than men. Pathological findings are usually absent, although in some patients, anatomical changes such as adhesions in the region of gasserian ganglion have been described. Because the disorder is paroxysmal in nature, antiepileptic drugs have been tried and are often found to be effective in alleviating the pain or stopping the episodes.

The first choice drug in the treatment of trigeminal neuralgia is carbamazepine in a dose of 200 mg 3–6 times daily.[10] The patient should start with a lower dose and increase it until the pain episodes are eliminated. A beneficial effect is often seen the day after onset of therapy. Carbamazepine blood levels of 6–12 µg/ml are usually seen in patients whose symptoms have been alleviated. Phenytoin in doses of 300 to 600 mg daily has considerably reduced the severity of pain and the frequency of episodes in many patients. Complete relief, however, is rarely achieved with phenytoin. It serves as a second choice drug for patients with hypersensitivity to carbamazepine.

Analgesics are of some benefit, but because of the fleeting nature of the episodes, are rarely satisfactory. In cases refractory to antiepileptic drugs, alcohol injections of the involved nerve branch may produce relief. After several months following the injection, the pain episodes tend to recur. Surgical retroganglionic section, which usually relieves the pain but leaves the patient with a numb face in the most severe cases, may be necessary.[22]

Side effects related to dose and high blood level are similar for carbamazepine and phenytoin, and include blurred vision, nystagmus, unsteadiness, and sedation. Skin rashes may be caused by either drug. Blood counts should be monitored because bone marrow depression has been caused by carbamazepine with occasional fatalities, particularly in elderly patients.

Glossopharyngeal neuralgia is characterized by episodic pain in the branches of that nerve. The condition is generally rare and may also be relieved by carbamazepine or phenytoin.

Postherpetic Neuralgias

Following herpes zoster infection, some patients develop postherpetic neuralgia. The pain is usually continuous rather than episodic, has a burning or tingling quality, and may be quite severe. Treatment with antiepileptic drugs is rarely beneficial in this condition. Some relief can be obtained with analgesics such as propoxyphene, pentazocine, or codeine. The effect of analgesics can be supported or potentiated with tranquilizers. Diazepam 5 to 20 mg daily, chlordiazepoxide 10 to 30 mg daily, or chlorpromazine 100 to 500 mg daily have been helpful in this respect. Spontaneous improvement may occur after several months in some patients, in others, the pain may continue for longer periods of time. In the latter group of patients, depression may develop and contribute to the discomfort. Imipramine, amitriptyline, or doxepin have been of benefit in such cases.[22]

Atypical Facial Pain

Patients with atypical facial pain have periods of pain in various areas of face, head, or neck which may last for hours or days. There are usually no trigger zones or precipitating factors such as tactile or thermal stimulation. Drug therapy is generally unsatisfactory in this condition. Limited or transient alleviation may be achieved with antiepileptic drugs, tranquilizers, analgesics, anti-migraine drugs, and placebos, which indicate the primary suggestive value of such treatments. Depression and delusional psychoses are frequent among patients with atypical facial pain, and those patients may benefit from anti-depressant or electroshock therapy.[22]

REFERENCES

1. AELLIG WH, NUESCH E: Comparative pharmacokinetic investigations with tritium-labeled ergot alkaloids after oral and intravenous administration in man. Int J Clin Pharmacol 15: 106–122, 1977.
2. ANTONY M, LANCE JW: Current concepts in the pathogenesis and interval treatment of migraine. Drugs 3: 153–182, 1972.
3. BIANCHINE JR, FRIEDMAN AP: Metabolism of methysergide and retroperitoneal fibrosis. Arch Intern Med 126: 252–254, 1970.
4. DIAMOND S, MEDINA JL: Double-blind study of propranolol for migraine prophylaxis. Headache 16: 24–27, 1976.
5. FANCIULLACCI M, GRANCHI G, SICUTERI F: Ergotamine and methysergide as serotonin partial antagonists in migraine. Headache 16: 226–231, 1976.
6. FORSSMAN B, HENRIKSSON KG, JOHANNSSON V, LINDVALL L, LUNDIN H: Propranolol for migraine prophylaxis. Headache 16: 238–245, 1976.
7. FOSTER JB: Migraine, traditional uses of ergot compounds. Postgrad Med J 52 (suppl. 1): 12–14, 1976.
8. FOZARD JR: The animal pharmacology of drugs used in the treatment of migraine. J Pharm Pharmacol 27: 297–321, 1975.
9. GRAHAM JR: Cardiac and pulmonary fibrosis during methysergide therapy for headache. Am J Med Sci 254: 23–34, 1967.

10. Killian JM, Fromm GH: Carbamazepine in the treatment of neuralgia. Use and side effects. Arch Neurol 19: 129–136, 1968.
11. Lance JW: The mechanism and management of headache. Butterworths, London, 1973.
12. Lance JW, Anthony M: Clinical trial of a new serotonin antagonist BC105 in migraine. Med J Austr 1: 45, 1968.
13. Lance JW, Anthony M, Sommerville B: Comparative trial of serotonin antagonists in the management of migraine. Br Med J 2: 327–330, 1970.
14. Meier J, Schreier E: Human plasma levels of some anti-migraine drugs. Headache 16: 96–104, 1976.
15. Mellander S, Nordenfelt I: Peripheral and circulatory effects of dihydroergotamine. Postgrad Med J (suppl 1) 52: 17–20, 1976.
16. Ostfeld AM: A study of migraine pharmacotherapy. Am J Med Sci 241: 192–198, 1961.
17. Pearce J: Hazards of ergotamine tartrate. Br Med J 1: 834–835, 1976.
18. Pedersen E, Moller CE: Methysergide in migraine prophylaxis. Clin Pharm Ther 7: 520–526, 1966.
19. Schmidt R, Fanchamps A: Effect of caffeine on intestinal absorption of ergotamine in man. Europ J Clin Pharmacol 7: 213–216, 1974.
20. Sicuteri F: Hypothesis: Migraine, a central biochemical dysnociception. Headache 16: 145–159, 1976.
21. Slugg PH, Kankel RS: Complications of methysergide therapy. JAMA 213: 297–298, 1970.
22. Taverner D: Drug treatment of cranial neuralgias. In: Handbook of Clinical Neurology. Eds: PJ Vinken, GW Bruyn. North Holland Publishing Co, Amsterdam. pp 378–401, 1968.
23. Walle T, Conradi EC, Walle UK, Fagan TC, Gaffney TE: The predictable relationship between levels and dose during chronic propranolol therapy. Clin Pharmacol Ther 24: 668–677, 1978.
24. Waters WE: Controlled clinical trial of ergotamine tartrate. Br Med J 2: 325–327, 1970.
25. Weber RB, Reinmuth OM: Treatment of migraine with propranolol. Neurology 22: 366–369, 1972.

8

Nervous System Complications With Systemic Metabolic Disorders

INTRODUCTION

The human central nervous system is adversely affected by a wide variety of metabolic disorders. When metabolic disorders are acute, they usually produce some degree of global neurologic dysfunction manifested as encephalopathy. When they are chronic, the cerebral hemispheres are affected, but in addition the peripheral nervous system frequently becomes involved. Among the common metabolic disorders that produce encephalopathy are diabetes with diabetic coma or hypoglycemia, hepatic disease, hypothyroidism, hypo- and hypercalcemia, adrenal cortical deficiency, amino acidemias, and drug-induced encephalopathy. The more common peripheral neuropathies associated with metabolic disease include nutritional deficiencies, alcoholic neuropathy, diabetes, the porphyrias, renal failure, and the ingestion of toxins. The effect of all these etiologies is to decrease the metabolism of neurons resulting in reduced axon flow and reduced neuro-transmitter production among other abnormalities. Encephalopathy and peripheral neuropathy are two nervous system changes associated with metabolic disorders.

METABOLIC ENCEPHALOPATHY

Diabetic Coma with Ketoacidosis

The most frequent encephalopathy associated with diabetic ketoacidosis is diabetic encephalopathy or coma. The clinical situation is characterized by varying degrees of either lethargy, stupor, or coma in individuals known to be diabetic, usually taking insulin, and in whom laboratory examination shows elevated levels of blood sugar, a reduction in serum pH, a reduction of plasma bicarbonate concentration, and generally some degree of dehydration.[37,5,23] The dehydration is due to severe osmotic diuresis related to the high blood glucose levels and the high excretion of glucose in urine. The dehydration is associated with loss of electrolytes as well as loss of water.

Treatment is directed towards lowering the blood sugar with insulin, correction of the dehydration with intravenous fluids, and correction of acidosis with bicarbonate. Insulin should be administered rapidly and be given as a soluble insulin.[5] The insulin dose should be at least 50 units initially, given intravenously. Following the initial dosage, doses of 10 to 20 units are given frequently, every 2 to 4 hours, until there is an appreciable fall of blood sugar to below 200 mg per 100 ml of plasma. Dehydration should be treated as rapidly as possible, frequently requiring 1 to 3 liters of fluid. Generally, fluid without glucose is used, but there is some danger in using isotonic saline because patients generally have lost more water than electrolytes. If available, hypotonic saline with a concentration of salt at .45 percent is useful. Potassium may be added to the intravenous solution in the amount of 10 milliequivalents per liter. The serum levels of potassium should be followed carefully during the treatment phase as well as blood pH and serum bicarbonate. Bicarbonate is generally used if the pH is extremely low, but is not necessary with mild reductions in pH. For patients in coma, 5 to 10 liters of fluid may frequently be required over the first 12 hours. Dextrose solutions can be substituted for saline when the blood sugar is brought under control and is approaching near normal levels. Patients with diabetic encephalopathy are frequently in jeopardy because of difficulty in handling secretions, and often have accompanying vomiting with aspiration pneumonia. It is recommended in deeply comatose patients that the stomach be emptied with a naso-gastric tube, and the naso-gastric tube be left in place until clear evidence of absence of gastric atony can be obtained. Blood chemistries must be estimated frequently to provide adequate rationale for treatment. Because infection is often the cause of poor diabetic regulation leading to coma, it should be sought for assiduously, and suitable antibiotic given when infection is found.

Hypoglycemia in Diabetics

Mild hypoglycemia among patients with diabetes who are taking insulin is a relatively common occurrence, manifested by brief periods of hypoglycemic symptoms such as weakness, lightheadedness and sweating. Occasionally, such states can be marked, with a major and prolonged alteration in the level of consciousness and, occasionally, coma.[26] For patients with mild transient symptoms of hypoglycemia, regulation of the diet and insulin dose, or addition of sugar at the time of the symptoms, will generally correct the situation. When coma is believed to be caused by hypoglycemia, immediate intravenous administration of 50 ml of a 50 percent solution of glucose should be carried out.[23] This is frequently a life-saving procedure, and is a treatment which can be given on the basis of suspicion before an absolute diagnosis is made because the treatment is essentially harmless. Some physicians advocate the use of 1 mg of glucagon which will rapidly reduce increased blood glucose levels. Intravenous glucose should never be given without previously drawing a blood sample for a blood sugar level.

Hyperosmotic Coma

Some diabetic patients develop coma without evidence of acidosis and ketoacidosis.[11,20] The cause is usually markedly elevated blood sugar with a hyperosmotic state. Hyperosmotic states can also be found in patients who have diabetes insipidus or in patients who have lost massive amounts of fluid following burns or loss from the intestinal tract with diarrhea. When suspected, the condition can be quickly diagnosed by determining the level of sodium or the osmolality of plasma. It can be rapidly corrected by giving hypotonic saline solutions intravenously until the serum sodium and serum osmols are within normal range.

Hyperosmolar states should be carefully watched for in patients who are receiving concentrated tube feedings, and in patients who are stuporous for other reasons, and cannot indicate their need for fluid.

Hypo-osmotic Coma

Hypo-osmolality occasionally causes coma and delirium, most often related to excessive voluntary intake of water or abnormalities in the hormonal control of water balance, such as in diabetes insipidus.[2,8,10] Occasional patients receiving diuretics for the treatment of congestive heart failure or edema, which selectively eliminates electrolytes, will develop water intoxication.[16] Characteristic laboratory findings are a low serum sodium concentration and a decrease in the osmolality of serum[17] normal values of which are approximately 290 to 300 milliosmol per liter. The most effective means of treating hypo-osmolar states is the restriction of fluid intake, generally to 500 to 1000 ml per day, and adding 5 percent sodium chloride when serum sodium is excessively low.

Hepatic Encephalopathy

Markedly impaired liver function is frequently associated with depression in the level of consciousness and evidence of acute delirium with disorientation, clouding of mentation, anxiety, and often hallucinations and delusions.[35] Encephalopathy in hepatic disease has been related to the accumulation of neurotoxic substances in the blood which have not been metabolized in the liver. It has also been associated with high levels of blood ammonia and abnormalities in carbohydrate metabolism in neurons.[27] The increased number of neurotoxins which are not metabolized in the liver has been related to an average, or more than average dietary intake of protein.

Treatment has been directed toward reducing the intake of protein in the diet and reducing the metabolic products of bacterial action in the intestinal tract, which contributes to hepatic encephalopathy.[36] The reduction of bacterial activity in the intestinal tract has been found to be effective means of treatment. This is carried out by placing the patient on oral antibiotics, the most commonly used antibiotic is neomycin which is largely unabsorbed and excreted in the feces.[12] For patients with hepatic encephalopathy, neomycin is given in doses up to 3 to 5 grams per day in divided doses. This will effectively sterilize the intestinal tract. Neomycin has strong ototoxic properties, and with longterm administration, careful observations for evidence of hearing loss must be made. Sterilization of the gut with neomycin may also give rise to other infections. Opportunistic infections with fungi, such as Candida, may develop in the intestinal tract causing difficulties. Dietary protein should be greatly restricted in patients with hepatic encephalopathy by maintenance on glucose or lactose by mouth, or intravenous infusions. Medications, especially sedatives and tranquilizers should not be given during the period of acute encephalopathy, because of the inability of the liver to metabolize them. When patients with liver failure have gastrointestinal bleeding, laxatives and purges are frequently useful in eliminating the blood from the intestinal tract and reducing the chances of its absorption which further aggravates the encephalopathy. Lactulose which is a non-absorbable disaccharide and is fermented in the intestinal tract to form acetic and lactic acids has been useful in promoting diarrhea. The dose of lactulose required is sizable and up to 50 to 60 grams a day are needed to produce diarrhea.

Hypothyroid Encephalopathy

Patients with myxedema often exhibit a marked degree of intellectual slowing, sometimes lethargy and occasionally coma.[14,32,21] When suspected, the diagnosis can easily be made by measuring serum thyroxin which is generally found in extremely low levels, below 2 μg/100 ml. The serum protein-bound iodine is always abnormally low (below 2 μg/100 ml) as well. The clinical diagnosis can also be suggested by changes in skin texture, hair texture and tendon reflex changes. Treatment of patients with myxedema coma and encephalopathy is risky and even with treatment, the mortality is high. If there is hypothermia, the patient should be gradually warmed with blankets. If there is carbon dioxide retention, the patient should be placed on a respirator to provide good ventilatory exchange.[33] If there is evidence of failure of other endocrine systems such as the adrenal or pituitary, suitable replacement therapy should be given, especially cortisol. Thyroid hormones should be administered with caution, and the exact program of treatment with thyroxin is still under debate. In patients with coma treated by slow supplementation of thyroid, there has been a conspicuous lack of success in treatment, and a high mortality. Some successes have been reported by rapid return to normal levels of thyroxin which requires a sizable amount of L-thyroxin, up to 500 micrograms as an initial dose followed by 100 to 200 micrograms daily. Cardiac problems are serious in patients with myxedema and encephalopathy, and frequently, restoration of normal metabolism with thyroxin administration is associated with cardiac failure or myocardial infarction.

Hypoadrenalism or Adrenal Cortical Insufficiency

Very rarely patients with adrenal cortical insufficiency will have mental and personality changes suggestive of encephalopathy. Such patients frequently complain of asthenia, exhaustion, difficulty with mental effort, and often are found to be confused and irritable and may develop delusions, and sometimes coma. The diagnosis of adrenal cortical insufficiency is based on finding a lack of the usual response of the adrenal glands to stimulation with ACTH and a reduced plasma cortisol level to below 15 micrograms per 100 milliliters. When the diagnosis has been made, hydrocortisone should be given. If the patient is in coma, it should be given intravenously in amounts of 100 to 200 milligrams followed by intravenous saline with maintenance doses of 100 milligrams of hydrocortisone daily or twice a day. When the patient has returned to normal level of mental functioning and there is no longer evidence of encephalopathy, maintenance dosage of prednisone or hydrocortisone should be given regularly for the life of the patient, prednisone 5 to 8 milligrams a day or hydrocortisone up to 30 milligrams per day are adequate.

Other Causes of Metabolic Encephalopathy

Other less common causes of metabolic encephalopathy include hyper- and hypocalcemia. Among patients who exhibit hypercalcemia, carcinoma of the breast and occasionally hyperthyroidism are among the causative conditions.[24,18] Such patients will frequently complain of nausea, vomiting and headache, and at times show abnormalities in their level of awareness, with confusion and delusions.[24] Often the condition can be partially alleviated by a low calcium intake, an elevated phosphate intake and a high fluid intake. For seriously ill patients intravenous sodium phosphate in doses of 1–2 gm given over 8–10 hours is useful. When the calcium level falls, oral sodium phosphate may be used.[18] Calcitonin can be used to reduce serum calcium. Definitive long term management requires removal of parathyroid adenoma or carcinoma of the breast.

Hypocalcemia as a cause of metabolic encephalopathy, is largely a condition found in children. The most common reasons for its occurrence in adults are problems of the parathyroid gland with hypoparathyroidism.[1] When patients develop hypocalcemia they usually have some degree of tetany in peripheral muscles, and convulsions can occasionally be seen.[25] They may show manifestations of chronic loss of intellectual function with dementia.[15] When a diagnosis of hypocalcemia due to hypoparathyroidism is made, the patient should be treated with increased amounts of calcium in the diet in the form of calcium lactate from 2 to 6 grams per day. Treatment with calciferol may also be started.

Encephalopathies Associated With Congenital Enzyme Deficiencies   There are a number of very rare neurological disorders characterized by alterations in the plasma concentrations and the elimination of amino acids in the urine. These are largely diseases of children with a distinct hereditary basis. They are generally linked with some enzymatic deficiency in the usual metabolic pathways of amino acids. The most commonly encountered of such disorders is phenylketonuria.[29]

Phenylketonuria is almost always first detected in children. The usual clinical features are lack of intellectual development, hyperactive motor disturbances, sometimes unusual behavior in the form of agitation, and occasionally, seizures. The diagnosis is confirmed by demonstrating an elevated concentration of phenylalanine in the blood. Regular measurement of phenylalanine in the blood of newborn infants is now routinely done as a screening method to detect unsuspected instances of phenylketonuria, which if untreated leads to mental retardation. When the disorder is discovered, phenylalanine should be restricted from the diet. In view of the fact that phenylalanine is an essential amino acid, it cannot be totally excluded and care must be taken to be certain that whatever dietary intake of phenylalanine is required to maintain normal growth, also maintains a near normal blood level. With growth and increasing age, the requirements of phenylalanine decline.

Other extremely rare causes of metabolic encephalopathy largely limited to children are related to insufficient decarboxylation of branch-chain ketoacids. Branch-chain biochemical defects are manifested among infants by lack of proper milestone achievement and failure to thrive, often associated with hypotonia and convulsions.[30] When the diagnosis is made, branch-chain amino acids must be largely excluded from the diet for the life of the infant. Plasma concentrations of these branch-chain amino acids must be carefully monitored and correlated with adequate diet to allow for a normal growth.

Drug Induced Encephalopathy   Probably the most common cause of metabolic encephalopathy in the adult is the use of drugs which have an action on the central nervous system. These drugs include most analgesics, tranquilizers, narcotics, sedatives, and drugs which are designed to change mood.[9,31] All these agents probably have some effect on the metabolism of the neuron, the production of neurotransmitters and their usual release and uptake. If such drugs are taken for long enough periods of time, they are frequently the cause of alterations in intellectual capacity. If these changes are acute, the diagnosis is delirium, and if chronic, the diagnosis is dementia. Both are manifestations of metabolic encephalopathy. Frequently, the symptoms of an acute metabolic encephalopathy (delirium) and chronic metabolic encephalopathy (dementia) are only encountered after the patient stops taking the medication. Patients who are especially sensitive to the metabolic effects of these drugs on the nervous system, are those with a mild to moderate evidence of decline in intellectual capacity prior to the use of such agents. In an adult who shows evidence of acute delirium or chronic dementia, the possibility of a metabolic encephalopathy due to the drug intake should be the first diagnosis to be excluded. In the past, bromide was the most frequent cause of disorders and currently such agents as tranquilizers, sedatives, and mood elevators lead the list. When identified, these agents should be stopped and the patient supported through the period of acute delirium. During that phase, adequate attention to nutritional intake, prevention of self harm because of anxiety and fear, and restoration of reality or near normal levels of reality should be undertaken. This is best done by enlisting the help of family and friends to be with the patient at all times. Following the disappearance of the acute phase of the metabolic encephalopathy, the patients are frequently left with permanent and nonreversible evidence of intellectual impairment, dementia. This may be marked enough so that the patient is no longer able to adequately manage his own affairs; or may be so slight that in situations in which the environment is highly structured and protected, functioning at normal levels is possible. All patients who are believed to have a metabolic encephalopathy, should have a careful drug screen, even when there is no historical evidence of drug use of any sort. Patients with other illnesses such as congestive heart failure, pneumonia, fever, dehydration and a variety of systemic illnesses, which produce a degree of debility, are especially sensitive to the cerebral metabolic effects of the agents mentioned. Any change in the behavior of a patient while in the hospital undergoing treatment for any of these mentioned disorders, should be looked upon as a manifestation of drug induced metabolic encephalopathy and should be followed by investigation for and removal of the probable toxic agent.

PERIPHERAL NEUROPATHY

Peripheral neuropathy is one of the most common manifestations of inadequate or abnormal neuronal metabolism in man.[14] It is commonly associated with a wide variety of systemic diseases such as diabetes,[7,38,19,3] inadequate intake of vitamins,[40] intake of a number of toxins, renal failure, or a variety of inherited metabolic abnormalities.[39,13] In underdeveloped parts of the world, peripheral neuropathy is most commonly associated with inadequate nutrition and inadequate vitamin intake.

Diabetic Peripheral Neuropathy

A physician in practice will probably, most commonly encounter the peripheral neuropathy associated with diabetes. In general, this is an asymptomatic disorder evidenced during the physical examination and rarely if ever, complained of by the patient. During a physical examination, the physician may find absent tendon reflexes at the ankle and be able to demonstrate some fall off in the perception of vibratory sense or of position sense in the lower extremities. The group of signs is very frequent in elderly or late onset diabetics, and usually causes no functional difficulty. The condition, however, may be progressive with increasing loss of reflex activity, loss of knee jerks, and loss of other reflex functions involving the bladder and the bowel, and a major loss of sensory perception.

Advanced forms of diabetic neuropathy largely affect the sensory input at the junction of the dorsal root entry zone, producing changes in normal and important reflex function. Patients often have severe enough involvement to develop orthostatic hypotension, incontinence of urine, feces and impotence. It is believed that the cause of dorsal root damage is damage in small blood vessels supplying the dorsal route entry zone.

To date, none of the phenomena of diabetic neuropathy have been altered in their usual course or improved in any way by the more careful management of diabetes either by insulin or oral antidiabetic agents. Treatment is largely symptomatic for the advanced state where orthostatic hypertension and incontinence become a problem.

Patients with diabetes may also develop another form of neuropathy, namely asymmetrical diabetic neuropathy, which is largely a motor disorder with pain, loss of strength and muscle atrophy in various muscle groups throughout the body in an asymmetrical distribution. This condition is also known as abiotrophy. It appears to be clearly related to the diabetic vascular process involving the ventral motor roots or peripheral nerve. It is a distressing syndrome because of the pain and marked weakness. The abiotrophy may be reversible but the reversal does not seem to be clearly connected with a more careful management of diabetes.

Rarely, one may encounter a diabetic with asymmetrical advancing peripheral neuropathy suggestive of that seen with nutritional insufficiency. This was common in diabetics before insulin was available and was largely the result of marked nutritional failure related to the enormous caloric and vitamin loss associated with excessive glycosuria and poor general nutrition.

For every diabetic who develops any form of peripheral neuropathy, more careful attention must be given to the adequate regulation of diabetes, to make certain that adequate vitamin and a balanced caloric intake is maintained. Whether improved control requires insulin, sulfonylureas or biguanidines is a matter of experience and judgment of the individual physician in managing the patient.

Alcoholic Peripheral Neuropathy

Alcoholic peripheral neuropathy has been discussed in part under vitamin deficiency states. In the developed countries, it is one of the most common causes of peripheral neuropathy. It is believed that the neuropathic dysfunction is not related primarily to the toxic effects of the alcohol itself, but to the lack of caloric intake and to the lack of associated necessary vitamins with the vitamin-free carbohydrate, alcohol. Treatment is always directed toward stopping the ingestion of alcohol, giving of an adequate diet, and supplementing the usual vitamin intake.

Characteristically, the peripheral neuropathy begins in the most distal parts of the body, usually in the feet. The condition first involves the largest nerve cells in the body, those that arise in the dorsal ganglia and supply the tendon and movement receptors in the great toe.[6] It is believed that these very large neurons are most susceptible to metabolic abnormalities due to disturbances of axonal flow with metabolic deficiencies. The condition generally develops symmetrically in both legs and progresses gradually. Involvement begins with the feet, then the legs. When the distance between the dorsal route ganglia or the anterior horn cell to the site of the level of neuropathy in the legs equals that distance from the cervical cord to the large joints in the hand, the condition appears in the upper extremities. If it goes untreated, other long nerves in the body will become involved, including the recurrent laryngeal nerve with the development of hoarseness. Characteristic symptoms are those of weakness, sensations of numbness, burning pain in the feet, pain and soreness in the parts involved. On examination, there is generally weakness, loss of muscle substance, loss of deep tendon reflexes, loss of perception to sensory modalities such as touch, pinprick, vibration and position sense, and a hyperalgesia in those areas which may be nearly anesthetic to pinprick when pressure is applied to muscle, tendon or joint. When the disease is recognized, improvement can easily be followed by the regression of these symptoms and signs, which may take as long as 6 to 8 months following the reversal of an inadequate diet and an inadequate vitamin intake. This curiously parallels the probable time taken for restoration of normal axonal flow and the time needed for normal axonal metabolic products to reach the peripheral portions of the axon. For treatment schedules, which are to include thiamine and niacine, see *Vitamin deficiencies.*

MYOPATHIES

A large number of myopathies are encountered in neurological practice. Endocrine myopathies may be encountered in hyperthyroidism, hypothyroidism, Cushing's disease, acromegaly and hypopituitarism. Generally, in all of these conditions, myopathy is rarely the presenting syndrome of the disorder and adequate treatment of these particular endocrine abnormalities leads to improvement of the myopathy.

Periodic Hypokalemic Paralysis

Periodic hypokalemic paralysis is a rare hereditary disorder which usually begins in childhood or early adolescence and is characterized by episodic periods of weakness or paralysis. It may be precipitated by sleep, excessive activity and sometimes by excessive intake of carbohydrates.[22] The diagnosis is usually easily established in patients who become generally weak or paralyzed and have extremely low levels of serum potassium. The disorder can be frequently quickly corrected by the use of oral or intravenous potassium chloride to overcome the serum hypokalemia. Serum potassium levels must be carefully followed during treatment, especially intravenous treatment. Enough potassium must be given to restore levels to normal. Prevention of this disorder is sometimes possible by the regular use of potassium chloride when symptoms of weakness appear.

Occasionally, patients with episodic paralysis will have hyperkalemia. In general, this condition is rarely disabling enough to require major treatment efforts. It can often be brought under control by the use of diuretics which promote potassium loss such as hydrochlorothiazide.[22]

Other myopathies are uncommon and difficult to treat. The most common of them are hereditary in nature, such as muscular dystrophy, and nothing to date has been found to be of use in halting the progressive nature of such conditions.

REFERENCES

1. ALBRIGHT F, REIFERSTEIN EC: The parathyroid glands and metabolic bone disease. Williams and Wilkins. Baltimore, 1948.
2. ARIEF AI, LLACH F, MASSEY SG: Neurological manifestations and morbidity of hyponatremia, correlation with brain water and electrolytes. Medicine 15, 1976.
3. ASBURY AK: Proximal diabetic neuropathy. Ann Neurol 2: 179–180, 1977.
4. ASHER R: Myxedematous madness. Brit J Med 2:555, 1949.
5. BARCHUS H: National management of diabetes. Univ Park Press. Baltimore, 1977.
6. BEHSEM F, BUCHTHAL F: Alcoholic neuropathy: clinical electrophysiological and biopsy findings. Ann Neurol 2: 95–110, 1977.
7. BRADLEY WG: Disorders of Peripheral Nerves. Blackwell Scientific Publications, Oxford, 1974.
8. BRISMAN R, CHUTORIAN AM: Inappropriate antidiuretic hormone secretion. Arch Neurol 23: 63, 1970.
9. CARNEY MWP: Five cases of bromism. Lancet 2: 523, 1971.
10. CARTER NW, RECTOR FC, SELDIN DW: Hyponatremia in cerebral disease resulting from the inappropriate secretion of antidiuretic hormone. New Eng J Med 264: 67, 1961.
11. DANOWSKI TS, NABARRO JDN: Hyperosmolar and other types of nonketotic acidotic coma in diabetes. Diabetes 14: 162, 1965.
12. DAWSON AM, McLAREN J, SHERLOCK S: Neomycin in the treatment of hepatic coma. Lancet 2: 1263, 1957.
13. DYCK PJ: Peripheral neuropathy in the nervous system, Tower DB, (ed) The Clinical Neurosciences. Raven Press. New York, 1975.
14. DYCK PJ, THOMAS PK, LAMBERT EH, (eds) Peripheral Neuropathy Vol. I, Vol. II. WB Saunders Co. Philadelphia, 1975.
15. ERANT D: Idiopathic hypothyroidism presenting as dementia. Brit Med J 1: 429, 1974.
16. FICHMAN MP, VORHERR H, KLEEMAN CR, TELFER N: Diuretic-induced hyponatremia. Ann Int Med 75:853, 1971.
17. FISHMAN RA: Neurological manifestations of hyponatremia in Handbook of Clinical Neurology. Vinker PJ, Bruyn GS (eds) 28. North Holland Publishing Co. New York, 1976.

18. FRAME B: Neuromuscular manifestations of parathyroid disease, in Handbook of Clinical Neurology. Vinker PJ, Bruyn GW (eds). North Holland Publishing Co. New York, 1976.

19. GARLAND H: Neurological Complications of Diabetes Mellitus: Clinical Aspects Proc R Soc Med 53:137, 1960.

20. GERICH JE, MARTIN MM, RECANT L: Clinical and metabolic characteristics of hyperosmolar nonketotic coma. J Neurophysiology 12: 173, 1971.

21. GREENE RAYMOND: The thyroid gland: Its relationship to neurology in Handbook of Clinical Neurology. Vinker PJ, Bruyn GW (eds). North Holland Publishing Co. New York, 1976.

22. GRIGGS RC: The myotonic disorders and periodic paralysis. In: Advances in Neurology, Vol. 17. Griggs, RC (ed). Raven Press, New York, pp 143–149, 1977.

23. JOSLIN EP: Treatment of diabetes mellitus. Lea & Febiger, Philadelphia, 1959.

24. KARPATE G, FRAME B: Neuropsychiatric Disorders in Primary Hyperparathyroidism. Arch Neurol 10: 387, 1964.

25. KUGELBERG E: Neurologic mechanisms for certain phenomena in tetany. Arch Neurol and Psych 56: 507, 1946.

26. LAWRENCE FE, MEYER A, NEVINS S: The pathological changes in the brain in fatal hypoglycemia. Quart J Med 11: 181, 1942.

27. LEAR EA, SHERLOCK S, SUMMERSKILL WHJ: Blood amonia levels in liver disease. Lancet 11: 836, 1955.

28. LUCAS CP, GRANT N, DAILY WJ, REAVEN GM: Diabetic coma without ketoacidosis. Lancet 1: 75, 1963.

29. MENKES JH, KOCH R: Phenylketonuria in Handbook of Clinical Neurology. Vol. 29. Vinker PJ, Bruyn GW (eds). North Holland Publishing Co. New York, 1976.

30. MOSER HW: Maple syrup urine disease. (Branched chain ketonuria) in Handbook of Clinical Neurology. Vol. 29. Vinker PJ, Bruyn GW (eds). North Holland Publishing Co. New York, 1976.

31. MURRAY RM, GREENE JG, ADAMS JH: Analgesic abuse and dementia. Lancet 2: 242, 1971.

32. NICKEL SN, FRAME B: Neurologic manifestations of myxedema. Neurology 8: 511, 1958.

33. NORDQUIST P, DHUNER KG, STEINBERG K et al: Myxedema coma and CO_2 retention. Acta Med Scand 166: 189, 1960.

34. Brain Dysfunction in Metabolic Disorders, Plum F, (ed). Assoc for Research in Nervous and Mental Disease Vol. 52. Raven Press. New York, 1979.

35. PLUM F, HINDFELT B: The neurological complications of liver disease in Handbook of Clinical Neurology. Vinker, PJ, Bruyn GW, (eds). North Holland Publishing Co. New York, 1976.

36. PLUM F, POSNER J: Diagnosis of stupor and coma. 2nd ed. FA Davis, Philadelphia, 1972.

37. RENOLD AE, STAUFFACHER W, CAHILL GF Jr: Diabetes mellitus in the metabolic basis of inherited disease. Stanbury JB, Wyngaarden JB, Friedrickson DS (eds). McGraw-Hill. New York, 1972.

38. RUNDLES RW: Diabetic Neuropathy, General Review Report of 125 Cases Medicine. 24: 111, 1945.

39. SIMPSON JA: The neuropathies in modern trends in neurology, Williams D (ed). Butterworths, Washington, 1962.
40. SPILLANE JD: Nutritional Disorders of the Nervous System. E & S Livingston. Edinburgh, 1947.
41. VICTOR M, ADAMS RD, COLLINS GH: The Wernicke-Korsakoff Syndrome. FA Davis & Co. Philadelphia, 1971.
42. WOLFF HG, CURRAN D: Nature of delirium and allied states. Arch Neurol Psychiat: 1175, 1933.

FURTHER READING

VICTOR M, ADAMS RD, COLLINS GH: The Wernicke-Korsakoff Syndrome. FA Davis & Co. Philadelphia, 1971.
PLUM F, (ed) Brain Dysfunction in Metabolic Disorders, Assoc for Research in Nervous and Mental Disease Vol 52 Raven Press, New York 1979.
WOLFF HG, CURRAN D: Nature of Delirium and Allied States Arch Neuro and Psych: 1175–1234, 1933.

9
Vitamin Deficiencies

With the development of knowledge of the biochemistry of vitamins and their role in human metabolism, a number of neurological conditions have been recognized as related to deficiencies for a particular vitamin or a number of vitamins. The epidemiology of neurologic conditions related to vitamin deficiency is largely related to an inadequate intake of specific vitamins, such as in situations of starvation and deprivation, or the use of particular nutrients which supply an adequate caloric intake but have no, or insufficient accompanying natural vitamins. The most common situation encountered in developed countries in the latter instance is chronic alcoholism. The first neurological disorder which was clearly connected with an inadequate intake of a substance, ultimately recognized as a vitamin (nicotinic acid), was pellagra. Later the relationship of thiamine to peripheral neuropathy was recognized and following

Table 9-1 / Vitamin Deficiencies

Vitamin	Daily requirement	Deficiency states occur at:
Niacin	4.4–6 mg/1000 K calories daily	Below 4 mg/1000 K cal.
Tryptophan	60 mg/100 K calories daily	Below 50 mg/1000 K cal.
Thiamine	.5 mg/1000 calories day	Below .2 mg/1000 K cal/day
Pyridoxine	1.2 mg/day	
Cyanocobalamin	1 μg per day	Serum Concentration below 100 pg/ml

that, the role of vitamin B-12, cyanocobalamin, and its lack in the genesis of subacute combined degeneration of the spinal cord. More recently, the role of pyridoxine, folic acid and calciferol have been elaborated and their connection with neurological disorders described. All of the substances now classified as vitamins are necessary for proper neurological function. In most instances neurological defects, when they occur, are usually related to deficiencies in more than one of these vitamins. In a few neurologic disorders, there are rather specific syndromes which seem to be related to a deficiency of one specific vitamin.

NICOTINIC ACID DEFICIENCY

Pellagra with its triad of diarrhea, dermatitis and dementia was formerly a common neurological syndrome encountered in large numbers in southern parts of the United States where diet was largely dependent on corn, and sporadically in areas of poor and inadequate nutritional intake in large sections of the world.[14] Ultimately, its cause was recognized as a lack of niacin or nicotinic acid. Niacin is supplied in the diet as nicotinic acid and can in part, be formed in the human organism by metabolism from tryptophan. Neurological syndromes are usually connected with deficiency of both nicotinic acid and tryptophan due to inadequate intake of the vitamin and the amino acid in the diet. The role of nicotinic acid has been identified and in the human organism, it becomes part of two coenzymes, diphosphopyridine nucleotide and triphosphopyridine nucleotide. Rarely, nicotinic acid deficiency is associated with malabsorption. The vitamin is readily absorbed from all portions of the intestinal tract. Daily requirements of nicotinic acid are believed to be in the range of 9 to 30 mg per day, or 4.4 mg niacin per 1000 calories. Nicotinic acid deficiency with pellagra in developed countries is now a sporadic occurrence and is usually related to dietary insufficiency or improper dietary habits.[12]

When dementia is identified as being due to nicotinic acid deficiency, the dose of nicotinic acid to correct the situation should be large and it is recommended that upwards of 100 mg daily should be given by mouth.[14] Nicotinamide is preferable to nicotinic acid as the latter frequently produces vasodilation, especially of the head and neck, which is uncomfortable for the patient. High doses of nicotinic acid or nicotinamide should be given for several months even with an improved dietary regimen, in order to correct the deficiency. Frequently, patients with dementia due to nicotinic acid deficiency take several months to show much in the way of restoration of normal intellectual capacity.

THIAMINE DEFICIENCY

Thiamine is probably the most widely known vitamin connected with neurological dysfunction and neurological abnormality. Deficiencies in thiamine intake have been associated with peripheral neuropathy (Beriberi), Wernicke's syndrome and its accompanying Korsakoff's psychosis.[12] A number of situations have been associated with thiamine deficiency including inadequate dietary intake, protracted vomiting, malabsorption and untreated disease of the large intestine. Daily requirements of thiamine are based on the caloric intake especially the amount of calories derived from carbohydrates.[7] For each thousand calories in the diet derived from carbohydrates, approximately .3 mg of thiamine is needed for proper carbohydrate metabolism. Thiamine deficiency is usually found when the daily intake of thiamine drops below .3 mg per 1000 calories. Thiamine is found in the body as thiamine pyrophosphate which is involved in the enzymic decarboxylization of alpha-ketoglutaric acid, and in transketolation in the hexose monophosphate shunt.[2,5] When thiamine is absent from the diet or deficient, pyruvic acid accumulates in the body. Thiamine is absorbed from the intestine probably by a system of active transport which is saturated when the intake of thiamine exceeds 20 mg a day.

In situations where patients are acutely ill, such as with Wernicke's syndrome,[17] it is preferable to replace the thiamine parenterally, and up to 100 mg a day should be given intramuscularly or intravenously in intravenous fluids. Regular oral administration for maintenance therapy should be in the range of 10 to 15 mg a day. In situations where thiamine deficiency neuropathy or Wernicke's syndrome is evident, as in the case of chronic alcoholics or nutritionally deprived individuals, restoration of nervous system function is variable. Manifestations such as ocular palsy as seen in Wernicke's syndrome are rapidly corrected.[7] The mental state of clouding in delirium is less rapidly corrected. It may take several months for restoration of dysfunction due to peripheral neuropathy. Patients deficient in thiamine must also be treated with a properly balanced diet with an adequate protein and carbohydrate intake.

VITAMIN B-12 DEFICIENCY

The discovery of vitamin B-12 may be considered an epic piece of medical investigation.[12] Deficiency of the vitamin has been related to megaloblastic anemia and subacute combined degeneration of the spinal cord. Early observation showed that substances found in liver could, when given parenterally, reverse megaloblastic anemia and improve the spinal cord syndrome. Later, a substance was identified which was present in liver but was not absorbed by individuals with megaloblastic or Addisonian pernicious anemia, due to atrophic gastritis and lack of an intrinsic factor in the gastric secretion. Ultimately, the specific substance responsible for the deficiency, cyanocobalamin, was identified. It was found that Vitamin B-12 was not absorbed from the intestinal tract in the absence of the intrinsic factor. A number of other causes of inadequate vitamin B-12 intake have been determined, including atrophic gastritis, removal of large portions of the stomach for the treatment of ulcer or cancer, removal of portions of the small bowel which decreases absorption, or inflammatory conditions of the small bowel which impairs absorption.[15] Inadequate vitamin B-12 intake has also been shown to be related to tropical sprue and to the presence of an intestinal parasite *Diphyllobothrium latum* (broad fish tapeworm), which was believed to preferentially consume most of the vitamin B-12 in the diet, giving rise to deficiency.[8] Vitamin B-12 is needed for the conversion of methylmalonyl Co-A to succinyl Co-A. When deficiency occurs methylmalonic acid appears in the urine.[13] The exact role of vitamin B-12 in the metabolism of the central nervous system is not clear. It is clear, in patients who are deficient in this substance, that the nervous system begins to function inadequately, giving rise to combined systems disease of the spinal cord, impaired dorsal and lateral column function, at times, peripheral neuropathy, occasionally optic atrophy and frequently dementia.[4,18] Because vitamin B-12 deficiency involves both the central nervous system and the blood forming capacity in humans, the two conditions are rarely, if ever, seen apart although frequently the presenting feature of vitamin B-12 deficiency can at first be anemia, or at first peripheral neuropathy, or dementia.

Vitamin B-12 deficiency is recognized by determining the serum concentration of the vitamin. The normal levels of vitamin B-12 in humans are 200 to 800 picograms per milliliter of plasma. Inadequate absorption of vitamin B-12 can be tested by the administration of radioactive vitamin B-12 and determining the amount of the vitamin which passes into the serum.[11] In pernicious anemia, very small amounts of the labeled vitamin are absorbed. The absence of intrinsic factor can be confirmed by giving vitamin B-12 with intrinsic factor and measuring the increased absorption of vitamin B-12.

When identified, a patient should be treated with 100 μg of vitamin B-12, given intramuscularly daily for approximately a week, followed by injections of 100 μg at monthly intervals after that. Because absorption is limited, due to lack of intrinsic factor or by abnormality of the intestinal tract, vitamin B-12 must be administered parenterally indefinitely. Large oral doses of 1–3 mg per week have been effective in some patients. For those situations in which abnormality of the intestinal tract, such as tropical sprue, or infestation with a worm, is the cause of the deficiency, it can be corrected by addressing the primary condition and treating it appropriately.

PYRIDOXINE (VITAMIN B-6) DEFICIENCY

Pyridoxine occurs as pyridoxal phosphate. It is an essential coenzyme for a number of transaminases and decarboxylases and is involved in the gamma-amino-butyric acid shunt in which alpha-ketoglutaric acid is converted to succinate.[16] Deficiencies in pyridoxine are related to a number of disease states.[3,6] In infants, seizures have been related to pyridoxine deficiency states,[10] the latter appears to be a familial disorder in which large amounts of pyridoxine are required to sustain normal metabolism.[3] In adults, pyridoxine deficiency has been associated with peripheral neuropathy and occasionally optic atrophy. Deficiency has been related to inadequate intake, or intake of antagonists of pyridoxine, such as isoniazid, or malabsorption as is seen in diseases of the large and small intestines such as tropical sprue.[9] The most common symptoms of the peripheral neuropathy in pyridoxine deficiency come from the descriptions given of the condition as it occurred in Japanese prisoner-of-war camps during World War II, where most individuals with deficiency complained of intense burning in the feet, and when examined had evidence of peripheral neuropathy.[12]

When pyridoxine deficiency is recognized, the substance should be added to the diet in relatively sizeable doses exceeding the daily requirement of 2 mg by a factor of 10 to 20. In situations where it is necessary to give drugs which antagonize the action of pyridoxine such as isoniazid or penicillamine, large amounts of pyridoxine must be administered along with these agents to avoid peripheral neuropathy, and seizures.

FOLIC ACID DEFICIENCY

Deficiency in folic acid intake has been associated with a number of neurological disorders including peripheral neuropathy and probably dementia and organic brain syndrome. The exact relationship of folic acid deficiency in these situations is unclear but in one instance it has been related to the long-term use of anticonvulsants, such as phenytoin, which can be associated with peripheral neuropathy.[1] It is generally believed sensible for patients who have peripheral neuropathy from nutritional deficiency, to give folic acid with other vitamins and nutrients, and to give folic acid along with anticonvulsants to individuals who develop evidence of peripheral neuropathy. Patients on long-term anticonvulsants therapy who develop megaloblastic anemia, who have shown low levels of folate in their systems, should be given folic acid. It is a water soluble vitamin and an intake of 10 to 20 mg daily is adequate replacement therapy.

REFERENCES

1. BAYLISS EM, CROWLEY JM, PREECE JM, et al: Influence of folic acid on blood pheny-toin levels. Lancet 1: 62, 1971.
2. DREYFUS PM: Transketolase activity in the nervous system. Wohlstenholme GEW (ed) Thiamine deficiency: Biochemical lesions and their clinical signifcance. Boston Little Brown, 1967.
3. FRIMPTER GW, ANDELMAN RJ, GEORGE WF: Vitamin B_6 dependency syndromes. Am J Clin Nutrition 22: 794, 1969.
4. HOLMES JM: Cerebral manifestations of Vitamin B-12 deficiency. Brit Med J 2: 1394, 1956.
5. McCANDLESS OW, SCHENKER S: Encephalopathy of thiamine deficiency studies of intracerebral mechanisms. J. Clin. Invest. 47: 2268, 1968.
6. MUDD SH: Pyridoxine-responsive genetic disease. Fed Proc 30: 970, 1971.
7. PHILLIPS GB, VICTOR M, ADAMS RD, et al: A study of the nutritional defects in Wernicke's syndrome. The effect of a purified diet, thiamine, and other vitamins on the clinical manifestations. J Clin Invest 31: 859, 1952.
8. RICHMOND J, DAVIDSON SP: Subacute combined degeneration of the spinal cord in non-addisonian megaloblastic anemia. Quart J Med 27: 517, 1958.
9. ROSS RR: Use of pyridoxine hydrochloride to prevent isoniazid toxicity. JAMA 168: 273, 1958.
10. SCRIVER CR: Vitamin B_6-dependency and infantile convulsions. Pediatrics 26: 62, 1960.
11. SILBERSTEIN EB: The Schilling test. JAMA 208: 2325, 1969.
12. SPILLANE JD: Nutritional disorders of the nervous system. Livingstone, Edinburgh, 1947.
13. STADTMAN JC: Vitamin B_{12}. Science 171: 859, 1971.
14. SYDENSTRICKER VP: The history of pellagra, its recognition as a disorder of nutrition and its conquest. Amer J Clin Nutr 6: 409, 1958.
15. THOMPSON RB, UNGLEY CC: Megaloblastic anemia associated with anatomic lesions in small intestine. Blood 10: 771, 1955.
16. TOWER DB: Pyridoxine and cerebral activity. Nutrition Rex 16: 161, 1958.
17. VICTOR MD, ADAMS RD, COLLINS GH: The Wernicke-Korsakoff syndrome. Contemporary Neurology ed. (Plum, F and McDowell, FH) FA Davis, Philadelphia, 1971.
18. VICTOR M, LEAR AA: Subacute combined degeneration of the spinal cord. Am. J. Med. 20: 896, 1956.

10

Treatment of Malignant Gliomas

The prognosis for patients with malignant gliomas is invariably poor. If untreated, the patients often succumb within a few months, usually from the compromise of vital functions from increased intracranial pressure. Surgical intervention relieves the pressure, alleviates the pressure-related signs and symptoms, and prolongs life to some extent.[1,2] Data from a controlled randomized prospective study (see Table 10-1) indicates that the median survival time of patients with malignant gliomas after maximum feasible surgical resection is approximately 17 weeks. If radiation therapy was applied following the surgery, the median survival time was prolonged to 38 weeks. Combining chemotherapy with surgery and radiation added a few weeks to the median survival time, but more important, increased the percentage of long-term survivors. The percentage of patients surviving 18 months or longer among those receiving surgery and radiation alone was 5 percent; this was increased to 28 percent by the addition of chemotherapy. Similar results have been observed in some other studies. It thus appears that chemotherapy has a place in the treatment regimen of malignant brain gliomas.[3,4,5,6]

On theoretical grounds, complete cure of brain tumors with best currently available chemotherapeutic agents is not expected. Because of their systemic toxic effects,they can be given only in doses that cause a cell-kill smaller than the average regrowth rate of the tumor. As in the treatment of systemic malignancies, the use of several agents may be more effective than the use of a single chemotherapeutic agent. Among the drugs that have shown the most promise are nitrosoureas supported by procarbazine or vincristine. Corticosteroids are

Table 10-1 / Results of Randomized Studies Evaluating Postoperative Therapy of Malignant Gliomas

Study	*Treatment*			
	SURGERY	SURGERY AND RADIATION	SURGERY AND CHEMOTHERAPY	SURGERY, RADIATION, AND CHEMOTHERAPY
Walker and Gehan, 1972				
Median survival in weeks	17	38	25	41
18 months survival in percent	0	5	5	23
Walker and Strike, 1976				
Median survival in weeks	—	37	27	46
18 months survival in percent	—	7	6	28
Shapiro and Young, 1976; Shapiro, 1978				
Median survival in weeks	—	—	35	63
18 months survival in percent	—	—	6	44

often used concurrently as needed, mostly to alleviate the increased intracranial pressure.[4]

Nitrosoureas, 1,3-bis(2-chloroethyl)-1-nitrosourea (BCNU), 1-(2-chloroethyl)-3-cyclohexyl-nitrosourea (CCNU), and 1-(2-chloroethyl)-3-(4-methycyclohexyl)-1-nitrosourea (Me CCNU) belong to the category of antimetabolites. They penetrate the blood-brain barrier easily and act by interfering with the incorporation of carbon fragments into the purine ring, thus hampering the production of the building blocks of nucleic acids. Procarbazine also acts by inhibiting the biosynthesis of nucleic acids. Vincristine, on the other hand, is a mitotic inhibitor producing a metaphase arrest.

A reasonable treatment plan for a patient with malignant glioma would be the following:[3,4]

(1) After surgery, during which as much of the tumor is removed as is possible, radiation therapy is started. A total of 6000 rads are given over a 6 week period; of this, 4500 would be whole brain radiation, and 1500 directed to the involved hemisphere.

(2) Chemotherapy is started in the second week following the operation. If BCNU is used, 80 mg per square meter per day for 3 days is given intravenously and repeated every 5 to 8 weeks as tolerated. If CCNU is used, 50 mg per square meter per day is given orally on day 1 and day 15, then the patient is rested for a month, following which the CCNU cycle is repeated. If procarbazine is used as well, it is given orally in a dose of 75 mg per square meter per

day for 4 weeks to coincide with CCNU administration periods. If vincristine is used, the dose is 1 mg per square meter per day given intravenously at 15 day intervals to coincide with the BCNU or CCNU administration periods. Dexamethasone in doses up to 4 mg four times a day may be used if signs and symptoms of increased intracranial pressure occur. The dose may later be reduced gradually and continued at a lower level, if needed.

Side effects occur in almost all patients receiving the chemotherapy. The BCNU and CCNU cause leukopenia and thrombocytopenia which reaches a low point in 3 to 4 weeks and takes a week or 10 days to recover. This necessitates the rest periods between the treatment periods. Platelet transfusions are given when the platelet count falls below 20,000–50,000 or when there is bleeding. Nitrosoureas may also cause refractory thrombocytopenia and anemia, usually after prolonged administration. Impairment of liver functions may occur, manifested by elevated SGOT, SGPT, and alkaline phosphatase values. The main toxic effect of procarbazine is leukopenia. Vincristine spares the hematopoietic system, but often causes peripheral neuropathy manifested by paresthesias of the fingers and toes, decreased tendon reflexes, and occasionally foot-drop. With carefully selected schedules and timing of treatments, these side effects are usually not prohibitory in the majority of the patients.[3,4]

Since no total cure can be expected, one may question the wisdom of chemotherapy of malignant brain tumors in general at the present time. There is, however, the possibility of prolonging life by a year in some patients; thus it seems to be a reasonable alternative. As new agents develop, the outlook should improve in the future.

REFERENCES

1. BLOOM HJG: Combined modality therapy for intracranial tumors. Cancer 35: 111–120, 1975.
2. GOLDSMITH MA, CARTER SK: Glioblastoma multiforme—a review of therapy. Cancer Treatment Reviews 1: 153–165, 1974.
3. SHAPIRO WR, YOUNG DF: Chemotherapy of malignant glioma with CCNU alone and CCNU combined with vincristine sulfate and procarbazine hydrochloride. Transactions Amer Neurol Assn 101: 217–220, 1976.
4. SHAPIRO WR: Chemotherapy of nervous system neoplasm. In: Primary Intracranial Neoplasms. (eds): Sher J Ford D Spectrum Publications, New York, 1978 (in press).
5. WALKER MD, GEHAN EA: An evaluation of 1,3-bis(2-chloroethyl)-1-nitrosourea (BCNU) and irradiation alone and in combination for the treatment of malignant glioma. Proc Amer Assoc Cancer Res 13: 67, 1972.
6. WALKER MD, STRIKE TA: An evaluation of methyl CCNU, BCNU and radiotherapy in the treatment of malignant glioma. Proc Amer Assoc Cancer Res 17: 163, 1976.

11

Infections of the Nervous System

Henry Masur, M.D.,* and Henry W. Murray, M.D.*

Infections of the central nervous system (CNS) can rapidly cause devastating destruction. Prompt institution of appropriate therapy is essential for the preservation of neurologic function. Optimal management of infection is based on rapid diagnosis and urgent institution of treatment. Once the infectious process has caused cerebral edema with transtentorial herniation or major vessel thrombosis, antimicrobial therapy and neurosurgery do little to alter the poor prognosis. This chapter will deal with the pharmacologic management of CNS infections and relate management to pathophysiology.

GENERAL CONSIDERATIONS

When the diagnosis of a CNS infection has been established, effective management depends not only upon immediate institution of medical therapy but also diligent observation for any subsequent changes which may occur in the patient's clinical status. Specific attention must be given to avoiding damage due to increased intracranial pressure, eradicating the responsible microorganism, anticipating local and systemic complications of therapy, and treating the original source of infection. General supportive measures such as management of respiratory complications, electrolyte disturbances, cardiovascular dysfunction, and rehabilitation are essential for optimal care, but are beyond the scope of this chapter.

*Assistant Professor of Medicine, Divisions of Infectious Diseases and International Medicine, Cornell University Medical College, New York, New York.

Choice of Antimicrobial Regimen

When a CNS infection is suspected, the identity of the pathogen can often be established within minutes, and thus, definitive therapy can be started. For instance, a military recruit presenting with meningitis during a *Neisseria meningitidis* outbreak, who has gram-negative diplococci in his cerebrospinal fluid (CSF) can be treated immediately with penicillin. The physician can be virtually certain that the antimicrobial regimen is appropriate. In most situations, however, the definite identity of the responsible pathogen(s) cannot be established immediately, and presumptive therapy has to be given on the basis of what pathogens are most likely in a specific clinical situation. Whether the pathogen is known with certainty or not, empiric therapy is to be started based on likely pathogens, the choice of the specific antibiotic to be used should be based on the following considerations.[19,28]

First, antimicrobial agents must be chosen to which the known or suspected pathogens are susceptible. In some situations, the susceptibility of the pathogen can be presumed with certainty. For instance, *Streptococcus pneumoniae* or beta-hemolytic streptococci are essentially always susceptible to low concentrations of penicillin or chloramphenicol. With other organisms, the susceptibility pattern may be in doubt. For example, *Escherichia coli* can be either sensitive or resistant to ampicillin or chloramphenicol, but is almost always sensitive to gentamicin. When designing initial therapy, the susceptibility of suspected organisms to drugs should be estimated from published data with consideration given to unusual sensitivity patterns in the patient's community. When the causative organism is isolated, its susceptibility should be assessed by an agar diffusion method such as the Kirby-Bauer technique. If feasible, agar or broth dilution method should be used to quantitate the minimum inhibitory concentration (MIC) or the minimum bactericidal concentration (MBC) of the chosen antibiotic for the causative organism.

Second, the penetration of the antimicrobial agent into the CSF or brain parenchyma must be considered.[28] The *in vitro* susceptibility of a pathogen to a given antibiotic reflects the sensitivity of the organism to concentrations of antibiotic that must be attained at the site of infection. Many commonly used antibiotics such as the cephalosporins, aminoglycosides, and clindamycin penetrate the CSF poorly, if at all. Thus, even if the pathogen is exquisitely sensitive to these drugs *in vitro,* they are ineffective for the treatment of central nervous system infections. While few drugs penetrate well into normal meninges or brain parenchyma, inflamed meninges are quite adequately penetrated by penicillin and chloramphenicol. Several other antibiotics also penetrate inflamed meninges adequately (see Table 11-1).

Since agents which penetrate the CSF and brain parenchyma are available for most pathogens, administration of antibiotics into abscess cavities or into

Table 11-1 / Relative Penetration of Antimicrobial Agents Into the Central Nervous System

	In the Presence of Inflammation	
Antimicrobial Agent	Cerebrospinal Fluid	Brain Parenchyma
Aminoglycosides		
Gentamicin	Poor	?
Tobramycin	Poor	?
Amikacin	Poor	?
Amphotericin B	Poor	?
Cephalosporins		
Cephalothin	Poor	Poor
Cephaloridine	Fair	Fair
Chloramphenicol	Excellent	Excellent
Chloroquine	?	Excellent
Clindamycin	Poor	Poor
Erythromycin	Good	Good
Ethambutol	Good	?
5-Fluorocytosine	Good	?
Isoniazid	Excellent	?
Lincomycin	Good	Good
Miconazole	Poor	?
Penicillins		
Penicillin G	Good	Good
Ampicillin	Good	Good
Carbenicillin	Good	Good
Ticarcillin	Good	Good
Nafcillin	Good	Good
Oxacillin	Good	Good
Methicillin	Fair	Good
Pyrimethamine	Good	Good
Quinine	Poor	Good
Rifampin	Good	?
Sulfadiazine	Excellent	Excellent
Tetracycline	Fair	Fair
Vancomycin	Fair	?
Vidarabine	Good	?

the subarachnoid space is rarely indicated. Intrathecal therapy is important, however, in certain gram-negative bacillary and fungal meningitides.[23,34,43] Administration of antibiotics into the lumbar sac rarely provides adequate drug levels within the ventricles or over the cerebral hemispheres. To achieve adequate drug concentrations in these areas, drugs often have to be administered through a prosthesis implanted into the ventricle rather than by the lumbar route.[14,23] If an antimicrobial agent which is effective against the causative organism and which reliably penetrates the CNS is not available and intrathecal therapy must be used, the actual bactericidal levels in the serum and CSF should be determined early in the course of therapy, since multiple factors make predictions of levels unreliable.

Third, some pathogens may be relatively resistant to most individual antimicrobial agents, but a combination of drugs may show *in vitro* synergy, and thus provide adequate therapy. For instance, many Pseudomonas are relatively insensitive to gentamicin, and rapidly become resistant to carbenicillin when this drug is used alone. The sensitivity of Pseudomonas *in vitro* to the combination of gentamicin and carbenicillin is more than additive. Antibiotic synergy has been shown for many organisms including *Streptococcus faecalis, Staphylococcus aureus,* and *Pseudomonas aeruginosa.* Use of a synergistic combination of drugs can produce a clinical response not possible with single-drug therapy.[3]

Fourth, the relative advantage of using a bactericidal antibiotic rather than a bacteriostatic drug has not been clearly established. Usually a bactericidal drug is preferable. There is some evidence that bactericidal and bacteriostatic drugs should not be given simultaneously for meningitis, because in theory, the bacteriostatic agent prevents bacterial multiplication which is necessary for bactericidal action.[28] Bactericidal and bacteriostatic drugs may be used together when some unusual situations such as mixed infections necessitate such combinations.

Fifth, patient tolerance to specific antibiotic drugs must be considered. A history of hypersensitivity or other adverse reactions should always be inquired for, because in most situations, an alternative drug can be found if the patient is allergic to the drug of choice. The toxicity of each drug must be considered in the initial choice of the antibiotic, and watched for carefully during the entire course of therapy. In certain situations, potential or developing toxicity may require the use of an alternative drug. For instance, progressive thrombocytopenia occurring during chloramphenicol therapy may warrant switching therapy to ampicillin if the isolated organism was sensitive to both drugs. Common adverse effects of antibiotics are listed in Table 11-2.

Specified Microbial Diagnosis

Although CNS infections must often be treated presumptively in an effort to avoid rapid neurologic destruction, it is important to identify the specific pathogen for several reasons.

First, there are many infectious agents which can cause similar symptoms or a specific syndrome. Presumptive antimicrobial therapy may be completely ineffective for the less commonly encountered microorganisms. For instance, infectious causes of mass lesions in the brain include bacteria, mycobacteria,

Table 11-2 / Important Adverse Reactions to the Principal Antimicrobial Agents Used in Central Nervous System Infections*

Note: Hypersensitivity reactions may occur with any antimicrobial agent. They are specifically mentioned only when particularly prominent.

Antimicrobial Agent	*Adverse Reaction*
Aminoglycosides	
Gentamicin	*Nephrotoxicity*
Tobramycin	Ototoxicity—*Vestibular* and auditory
Amikacin	
Amphotericin B	*Nephrotoxicity*
	Chills, fever,
	Thrombophlebitis
	Anemia
Chloramphenicol	*Reversible bone marrow depression*
	Aplastic anemia
	"Gray baby" syndrome
	Optic and peripheral neuritis
Chloroquine	Corneal opacity, retinal damage
	Convulsions, headache
	Gastrointestinal irritation
	Hair and nail pigmentation
Erythromycin	*Thrombophlebitis*
Ethambutol	Optic neuritis
5-Fluorocytosine	Bone marrow depression
	Hepatotoxicity
	Gastrointestinal disturbance
	Headache, confusion, vertigo
Isoniazid	Peripheral neuritis
	Convulsions, psychoses
	Hepatitis
Lincomycin	Gastrointestinal disturbance
	Leukopenia, thrombocytopenia
Penicillins	*Hypersensitivity*
	Coombs positive hemolytic anemia
	CNS irritation
Ampicillin	Rash, diarrhea
Carbenicillin	Sodium overload
Methicillin	Nephritis
	Granulocytopenia
Nafcillin	Granulocytopenia
Oxacillin	Hepatotoxicity
Pyrimethamine	*Folic acid deficiency*
	CNS irritation
Quinine	Blood dyscrasia
	Cinchonism
	Hypotension

(continued)

Table 11-2 (*cont.*)

Antimicrobial Agent	Adverse Reaction
Rifampin	Hepatitis
	Leukopenia, thrombocytopenia
Sulfonamides	*Hypersensitivity*
	Agranulocytosis
	Hepatitis
	Crystalluria
Tetracycline	Thrombophlebitis
	Tooth enamel stains (children)
	Pseudotumor cerebri
	Fatty degeneration liver
	Azotemia
	Fanconi syndrome
Vancomycin	Thrombophlebitis
	Nephrotoxicity
	Ototoxicity

*Common reactions are italicized.

fungi, protozoans, and metazoans. Penicillin and chloramphenicol therapy would obviously be inappropriate for a tuberculoma or a cryptococcal or amebic abscess. Even among bacteria, the range of species responsible for meningitis or abscess is extensive. It is important to be certain that no bacteria are present which are resistent to the planned antimicrobial regimen. For instance, *Pseudomonas aeruginosa* meningitis requires specific therapy with a drug (an aminoglycoside) not ordinarily used for meningitis, and by a route (intrathecal) which would not usually be employed were the identity of the organism unknown.

Second, resistant strains of bacteria and fungi are being found in the community and in hospitals with increasing frequency. Therefore, the causative organism must be isolated so that its sensitivity to various antibiotics can be assessed.

Third, identification of the specific organism can give important clues about the origin of the infection or the presence of underlying disease. For instance viridans streptocoocal meningitis in a young patient with a diastolic heart murmur should suggest endocarditis.[41] Similarly cryptcococcal meningitis should suggest the possibility of an underlying metabolic or immunologic disorder such as diabetes or leukemia.[10]

Surgical Management

Surgical intervention is important to relieve increased intracranial pressure caused by mass lesions. It is also important to debride contiguous infections, to remove foreign bodies, and to repair mechanical sequelae of the inflammatory response. The need to debride contiguous infections such as chronic sinusitis, middle ear infections, or soft tissue suppuration is obvious if cure is to be achieved.[41] When infection occurs in patients with intracranial prostheses such as Ommaya reservoirs and ventriculo-atrial shunts, these foreign bodies usually must be removed for cure of the infection.[14,38]

Meningitis may be associated with sufficient inflammation to cause obstruction to CSF outflow: treatment of the resulting hydrocephalus may require a shunt for decompression. Patients with recurrent meningitis due to a traumatic or post-surgical CSF leak may need surgical repair.

The optimal timing of the neurosurgical procedure, and the precise technique to be used require extensive experience and expertise. When the need for such procedures appears likely, a neurosurgeon should be consulted promptly.

Medical Management of Cerebral Edema

The benefit of corticosteroid therapy for cerebral edema has not been unequivocally established.[19] The use of corticosteroids in specific infectious syndromes is discussed in subsequent sections. Experimental evidence and anecdotal experience suggest that in brain abscess, viral encephalitis, and tuberculous meningitis, cerebral edema and vasculitis may respond to corticosteroids. Whether these possible benefits outweigh the suppressive effect which corticosteroids have on the immune response is uncertain. An important role for corticosteroids in the management of central nervous system infections seems to be widely accepted only for brain abscesses.[36] The onset of the anti-inflammatory effect of corticosteroids requires at least 4 to 8 hours. Decadron 4 mg intravenously every 4–6 hours, or methyl prednisolone 60 mg every 4–6 hours are appropriate regimens.

Osmotic diuretics such as mannitol and glycerol can temporarily reduce intracerebral pressure by means of volume depletion. Mannitol should be given as a 20 percent solution, 1–2 gm/kg intravenously over 30–60 minutes. The use of osmotic diuretics is confined to brief, urgent situations in which transtentorial or uncal herniation must be prevented while the patient is prepared for surgery. They are not beneficial for long-term management due to the rebound increase of intracranial pressure which quickly occurs, and the systemic electrolyte imbalances which can result.

Anticonvulsant Therapy

Focal and generalized seizures can be caused by inflammation or irritation of brain parenchyma or the meninges. Anticonvulsant therapy is often used prophylactically when a brain abscess or subdural empyema is present or a craniotomy has been performed.[19] Anticonvulsant therapy is usually continued at least until the signs of active infection and radiologic evidence of any mass lesion have disappeared. Phenytoin is the drug of choice. A patient is usually administered 750–1000 mg of phenytoin orally in 3 or 4 divided doses over 24 hours. It can be administered intravenously, but it must be given slowly and the patient's electrocardiogram should be monitored during the infusion to avoid dysrhythmia. In an urgent situation such as status epilepticus, 1000 mg of phenytoin can be given intravenously in one bolus at a rate of 50 mg/minute. Determination of phenytoin levels is useful and helps to obtain optimal therapeutic levels (10–20 μg/ml). Phenobarbital (60 mg per day in divided doses) can also be given intramuscularly or orally but has the disadvantage of causing somnolence and thus obscures the patient's clinical status. An individual seizure can conveniently be treated with diazepam 5–10 mg given intravenously.

Conditions Predisposing to CNS Infections

Effective management of CNS infections frequently depends on recognition of cranial or systemic diseases which predispose to CNS infections. Common predisposing conditions are listed in Table 11-3. Some are amenable to surgical treatment such as suppurative sinusitis or mastoiditis. Endocarditis and pulmonary infections may be associated with CNS infection and are examples of distant infections. These may require therapy that goes beyond that necessary for the CNS infection alone. Immunosuppressive therapy predisposes patients to CNS infections and immunosuppressive agents may have to be discontinued in order to treat the CNS infection adequately.

Complications of CNS Infections

Table 11-4 lists the prominent complications associated with CNS infections.

Cerebral edema with uncal herniation and compression of the mid brain is the most serious.[9,41] Some of the acute effects of CNS infection such as altered levels of consciousness, paresis, cranial nerve palsy and seizures may resolve partially or totally with therapy particularly if they are primarily manifestations of mild cerebral edema. Some of the complications may be irreversible particularly if they are the result of severe arachnoiditis or arteritis or venous thrombosis resulting in cerebral infarction. Brain stem compression may be irreversible and is often a common cause of death with CNS infection.

Some complications may occur late in the course of the infection. Deterioration of the neurologic state with developing stupor or coma may be due to developing hydrocephalus resulting from obstruction of CSF outflow or be caused by meningeal exudates, brain abscess, subdural effusions or empyema.

Table 11-3 / Common Predisposing Causes of Central Nervous System Infections: Likely Pathogens and Presumptive Theory

Predisposing Cause	Likely Pathogens	Initial Antimicrobial Regimen*	
		First Choice	Alternative Regimen for Penicillin Allergic Patients
Non-penetrating Cranial Trauma			
Infection < 3 days after trauma	*Streptococcus pneumoniae*	Penicillin	Chloramphenicol
Infection > 5 days after trauma	*Staphylococcus aureus* Gram-Negative Bacilli	Nafcillin and Gentamicin and Chloramphenicol	Vancomycin and Gentamicin and Chloramphenicol
Penetrating Cranial Trauma			
Cranial Osteomyelitis Neurosurgery Diagnostic Procedures Entering the Subarachnoid Space Cranial or Spinal Defects Head and Neck Neoplasm	B-Hemolytic streptococci *Staphlococcus aureus* Gram-Negative Bacilli	Nafcillin and Gentamicin and Chloramphenicol	Vancomycin and Gentamicin and Chloramphenicol
Fracture of Cribiform Plate	*Streptococcus pneumoniae* *Haemophilus influenza* Anaerobes	Chloramphenicol	

CSF Rhinorrhea	*Streptococcus pneumoniae*	Penicillin	Chloramphenicol
Otitis	*Streptococcus pneumoniae* *Haemophilus influenza* *Staphylococcus aureus* Gram-Negative Bacilli	Nafcillin and Gentamicin and Chloramphenicol	Vancomycin and Gentamicin and Chloramphenicol
Sinusitis	*Streptococcus pneumoniae* *Haemophilus influenza* Anaerobes	Chloramphenicol	
Central Nervous System Prosthesis	*Staphylococcus epidermidis* Diphthroids Bacillus Species Staphylococcus Gram-Negative Bacilli	†	
Primary Extracranial Infection			
Pulmonary	*Streptococcus pneumoniae* Anaerobes	Chloramphenicol	
Biliary and Intestinal	Enterobacteriaceae Anaerobes	Chloramphenicol and Gentamicin	

(*continued*)

Table 11-3 (cont.)

Table 11-3 / Common Predisposing Causes of Central Nervous System Infections: Likely Pathogens and Presumptive Theory

Predisposing Cause	Likely Pathogens	Initial Antimicrobial Regimen*	
		First Choice	Alternative Regimen for Penicillin Allergic Patients
Primary Extracranial Infection (continued)			
Gynecologic	Enterbacteriaceae *Listeria monocytogenes* Anaerobes	Chloramphenicol and Gentamicin	
Skin and Cranial Cellulitis	B-Hemolytic Streptococci *Staphylococcus aureus*	Nafcillin	Vancomycin
Endocarditis	*Viridans streptococcus Staphylococcus aureus Streptococcus faecalis*	Vancomycin	
Altered Immune Response	*Listeria monocytogenes* Gram-Negative Bacilli *Streptococcus pneumoniae Neisseria meningitidis* *Cryptococcus neoformans*	Penicillin and Chloramphenicol and Gentamicin (Carbenicillin‡) (Amphotericin§)	

*When Gram's stain and counter immune electrophoresis of cerebrospinal fluid or pus is non-diagnostic. If the patient has received antimicrobial therapy in the recent past these recommendations may require modification.

†Therapy is often withheld pending bacteriologic diagnosis in stable patients. Gentamicin and Chloramphenicol may be used as the initial regimen in unstable patients.

‡Carbenicillin should be initial therapy in granulocytopenic patients.

§Initial therapy with Amphotericin B should be considered in moribund patients, or those deteriorating on antibacterial therapy.

Table 11-4 / Complications of Central Nervous System Infections

Acute Phase	Chronic Phase
Cerebral Edema ± Herniation	Focal Neurologic Defects
Cerebral Arteritis	Hemiparesis
Seizures	Cranial Nerve Palsy
Focal Neurologic Deficits	Psychiatric and Cognitive Dysfunction
Hemiparesis	Seizures
Cranial Nerve Palsy	Brain Abscess
Ataxia	Subdural Effusion or Hematoma
Cortical Blindness	Hydrocephalus
Venous Sinus Thrombosis	Mycotic Aneurysm
Psychiatric and Cognitive Dysfunction	Pituitary Insufficiency
Subdural Effusion or Hematoma	Arachnoiditis
Hyponatremia	

Seizures may first occur during convalescence. Pituitary insufficiency may not be apparent until the major neurologic manifestations are fully resolved.

A number of systemic complications can occur in any severely ill patient with central nervous system infection: they should be watched for prospectively. The most common are aspiration pneumonia, electrolyte imbalance, hyperglycemia, cardiac dysrythmia, gastrointestinal hemorrhage and disseminated intravascular coagulation.[9,41] These problems require the same careful monitoring and prompt therapy which patients with any type of devastating illness receive.

Commonly Used Antimicrobial Agents

The appropriate agents for specific types of CNS infections are discussed in the sections describing the various types of infections. The drugs of choice and feasible alternatives are also listed in Tables 11-3, 11-5 and 11-7. This section provides details concerning the pharmacology of the commonly used drugs, and other information important in their clinical use. The adverse effects of these drugs are listed in Table 11-2.

Antibacterial Agents

Chloramphenicol is a highly useful drug for the treatment of bacterial CNS infections due to its broad spectrum of antibacterial effect and its superior penetration of both the brain and meninges.[28,33] Chloramphenicol is a bacteriostatic agent which inhibits bacterial protein synthesis by acting at the 50s ribosomal sub-unit to suppress peptide bond formation.

Chloramphenicol is effective against a broad range of gram-positive and gram-negative organisms.[33] It is active against most of the common CNS pathogens, including *N. meningitidis, H. influenzae, S. pneumoniae,* most anaerobes, and many strains of *S. aureus, E. coli,* and proteus species. Like all antibiotics, penetration of chloramphenicol into the meninges and brain parenchyma is not completely predictable even in the presence of inflammation, but its penetration is superior to all other commonly used antibiotics. High serum levels are usually associated with good neurologic response. Although well absorbed orally, chloramphenicol should be administered intravenously for serious CNS infections. The adult dose is 0.5–2.0 gms given every six hours. Chloramphenicol is inactivated by hepatic conjugation and excreted in the urine. The dosage must be decreased in the presence of severe hepatic disease.

Because chloramphenicol inhibits mitochondrial protein synthesis in both bacterial and mammalian cells, it is invariably associated with a dose-related, reversible bone marrow depression. The hematocrit, white blood count, platelet count, and iron saturation should be monitored at least twice a week. The daily dose should be carefully adjusted on the basis of the MIC of the organism and the antibiotic levels measured in blood, CSF or pus. Serum levels should be maintained below 25 µg/ml to avoid the dose related reversible bone marrow toxicity. The use of chloramphenicol may be associated with a rare (one per 40,000 patients) idiosyncratic (non-dose related) marrow aplasia which is usually irreversible. Other adverse effects include encephalopathy, optic neuritis, mouth soreness, coagulopathy, and the "Gray Baby Syndrome". The rare association of chloramphenicol with idiosyncratic bone marrow aplasia should not prevent the use of this effective antibiotic for serious CNS infections.

Benzyl Penicillin (Aqueous Crystalline Penicillin G)   is a safe bactericidal antibiotic which penetrates well into the meninges and brain parenchyma.[28] It is highly active against several common CNS pathogens. Penicillin acts by interfering with the biosynthesis of the peptide chain cross links in bacterial cell walls. To be effective, penicillin is dependent on actively dividing bacteria. After exposure to penicillin, newly formed organisms are quite susceptible to osmotic lysis, though host defense mechanisms are probably also necessary for an adequate clinical response. Benzyl penicillin is highly effective against most strains of *N. meningitidis, S. pneumoniae,* and *Listeria monocytogenes.* Only a few *S. aureus,* group D streptococci, or gram-negative bacilli are sensitive to penicillin. Pentration of penicillin through the meninges and into the brain parenchyma is poor in the absence of inflammation. Although inflammation is associated with unpredictable penetration, high serum levels of penicillin are usually associated with substantial CNS concentrations and a good clinical response. There are seldom compelling indications to administer penicillin intrathecally. In the rare event that intrathecal therapy is necessary, no more than 20,000–30,000 units should be administered every 18–24 hours by the lumbar route in a volume of 10 cc of CSF or sterile saline, as intrathecal penicillin can cause encephalopathy, arachnoiditis and seizures. Less drug should be given into the ventricles or cisterna magnum. Penicillin may be inactivated by the host cell constituents of pus, and thus the bactericidal action of this drug is not reliable when gross pus is present.

The recommended regimen after an initial intravenous bolus of 5 million units is 24 million units per day by continuous drip, or 1 million units per hour. Since the half-life of penicillin is short (30 minutes), intervals between doses of more than one hour are not recommended. Penicillin is excreted by the kidneys, and dosage should be reduced in the presence of renal insufficiency. The use of penicillin is associated with few serious adverse reactions. Hypersensitivity is the most frequent, and its manifestations include anaphylaxis, serum sickness, urticaria, fever, and rash. Any history of hypersensitivity is an indication to use an alternate drug. The skin tests for hypersensitivity available to most physicians are not discriminating enough to be reliable. When there is a history of penicillin allergy, penicillin should be used only when no effective alternative is available and only after careful and rigorous hyposensitization. Nephritis and hemolytic anemia are rarely associated with penicillin therapy. Seizures can occur when the CSF concentration of penicillin is greater than 10 units/ml, seen sometimes when penicillin has been administered intrathecally or massive doses have been given in the presence of renal failure.

Ampicillin is a semisynthetic penicillin which differs from benzyl penicillin by virtue of its extended antimicrobial spectrum. It is active against both gram-positive and gram-negative cocci and gram-negative bacilli.[28] Its spectrum includes *N. meningitidis, H. influenzae, S. pneumoniae,* many anaerobes, and many *E. coli.* It is well suited for treatment of CNS infections in situations where non-specific therapy is begun while awaiting CSF culture results. The pharmacology of ampicillin is similar to benzyl penicillin, but its half-life is considerably longer. The administration of 2–3 g every four hours provides generally effective serum levels. Penetration into the CSF and brain parenchyma is comparable to that of penicillin, and is poor in the absence of inflammation, but adequate (though erratic) when inflammation is present. Intrathecal administration is rarely warranted. Adverse reactions are similar to benzyl penicillin, but skin rashes are more common.

Penicillinase Resistant Penicillins. Methicillin, oxacillin, and nafcillin are semisynthetic penicillinase (beta-lactamase) resistant penicillins useful for the therapy of CNS staphylococcal infections, as all penetrate the inflamed meninges. Nafcillin probably penetrates both inflamed and non-inflamed meninges better than methicillin.

Nafcillin and oxacillin are associated with fewer adverse effects than methicillin and generally are preferred. For CNS infection, high doses of nafcillin or oxacillin should be administered intravenously, 2 g every four hours. Nafcillin is associated with rare instances of nephritis, leukopenia, or phlebitis, and oxacillin may cause hepatic toxicity. Both are excreted primarily by the liver.

Carbenicillin and ticarcillin are semisynthetic penicillins which are useful when combined with an aminoglycoside in the treatment of certain CNS infections caused by gram-negative bacilli such as *Pseudomonas aeruginosa*. Carbenicillin diffuses well through inflamed meninges. Since the drug has a short half-life, 0.5 g/kg/day should be given intravenously in divided doses every four hours. Carbenicillin plus an aminoglycoside are frequently synergistic against *P. aeruginosa* and several other gram-negative bacilli. When high doses of carbenicillin are used, sodium overload must be watched for. In patients with renal insufficiency or sodium retention, ticarcillin can be used instead of carbenicillin since ticarcillin contains less sodium. Carbenicillin is usually not appropriate by itself for treatment of CNS infections due to the rapid emergence of resistance among *P. aeruginosa* strains and the lack of extensive clinical experience with gram positive infections.

Cephalosporins. In general, cephalosporins should not be used for CNS infections since penetration into the CSF and brain parenchyma is extremely poor.[34] CSF levels may be only 1 percent of simultaneously determined serum concentrations. Cephaloridine however, has been used in some situations, and effective levels have been found in brain abscesses and CSF. The profound nephrotoxicity of this drug makes it undesirable except in unusual and desperate situations.

Sulfonamides. Sulfadiazine, sulfadimidine, sulfamethoxazole, or sulfafurazole penetrate inflamed meninges well and can be highly effective for the treatment of sensitive *N. meningitidis*, *Nocardia asteroides* or *Toxoplasma gondii*. These drugs disrupt folic acid synthesis and are thus bacteriostatic. The emergence of resistant bacteria, especially *N. meningitidis*, *S. pneumoniae* and *H. influenzae* strains has limited the usefulness of sulfa drugs for bacterial infections. Chloramphenicol or a penicillin are almost always preferable for any bacterial CNS infection. Since sulfa drugs penetrate the CNS and since all Nocardia and Toxoplasma are sensitive to sulfa drugs, they are used for the treatment of CNS toxoplasmosis and nocardiosis. Co-trimoxazole, a fixed combination of sulfamethoxazole and trimethoprim, has not as yet had sufficient clinical trials to warrant its use as first-line therapy for any CNS infection except Nocardiosis.

Aminoglycosides have broad bactericidal activity against gram-negative bacilli. They act directly on the bacterial ribosomes to inhibit protein synthesis. Most gram-negative bacilli are sensitive to gentamicin and tobramycin, including most *P. aeruginosa,* Klebsiella-Enterobacter species, *Proteus* species, and *E. coli.* The toxicity of the aminoglycosides and their poor penetration into the CSF and brain parenchyma call for their careful and skilled use for those CNS infections caused by chloramphenicol and ampicillin resistant organisms.

Gentamicin and tobramycin are the most commonly used aminoglycosides because of their effective broad spectrum against gram-negative bacilli, and their less severe toxicity compared to other members of this group of drugs.[23,33,34] Intravenous administration of 3–5 mg/kg/day usually results in effective but non-toxic serum levels (6–12 μg/ml). Serum levels must be carefully measured and renal function closely monitored. The half-life of gentamicin is 2 hours, thus, the drug should be given at 6 hour intervals. The drug is excreted by the kidneys, and dosage must be substantially reduced in patients with impaired renal function. Penetration into the CSF is variable but usually poor. Intrathecal administration of preservative-free gentamicin or tobramycin (5–10 mg every 18–24 hours) is often necessary for gram-negative bacillary meningitis.[23,33,34] Since lumbar administration does not result in reliable gentamicin concentrations in the ventricles or over the cerebral hemispheres, intraventricular aminoglycoside administration may be necessary.[23] Gentamicin and tobramycin are probably equally effective against sensitive organisms. The initial choice between the two depends on the general sensitivity patterns in the community or hospital, and ultimately, the MBC of the specific pathogen. Amikacin, a newer aminoglycoside should be reserved for gentamicin and tobramycin resistant organisms.

The aminoglycosides are ototoxic and nephrotoxic. Vestibular rather than cochlear dysfunction is the more common manifestation of ototoxicity for gentamicin and tobramycin. Intrathecal administration of gentamicin or tobramycin can result in painful radiculitis.

Erythromycin penetrates the inflamed meninges sufficiently to be an alternate drug for infections caused by *S. aureus, S. pneumoniae,* and other streptococci if penicillin or chloramphenicol cannot be used. Erythromycin inhibits protein synthesis by binding to the 50s ribosomal sub-unit, and can be either bactericidal or bacteriostatic, depending on the nature of the microorganism. Intravenous administration of 1 g every six hours should be adequate for therapy, but this method of erythromycin administration may cause sclerosis and thrombophlebitis at the intravenous site.

Tetracycline   gradually enters both non-inflamed and inflamed CSF after intravenous administration. Use of this bacteriostatic drug should be limited to infections caused by organisms known to be quite sensitive to tetracycline and then only when more reliable alternate therapy is not available.

Lincomycin and Clindamycin.   Lincomycin attains sufficient levels in CSF and brain parenchyma to inhibit several organisms. It may be a satisfactory alternative antibiotic in the unusual situation when a penicillin or chloramphenicol cannot be used. Lincomycin, binds to the 50s sub-unit of bacterial ribosomes and suppresses protein synthesis. Most *S. pneumoniae* and *S. aureus* strains are sensitive to it. High doses—600 mg intravenously every 6 hours—should be used. Untoward reactions are unusual, but include neutropenia, thrombocytopenia, hypersensitivity, and hepatotoxicity. Since clindamycin does not penetrate the meninges as well as lincomycin, there is no indication for its use for CNS infection.

Vancomycin   is a bactericidal drug which is active against most aerobic gram-positive cocci. It penetrates inflamed meninges adequately.[20] For CNS infections, 500 mg intravenously every 6 hours should be employed. Limited data suggest that this drug can be a useful alternative to penicillin or chloramphenicol in certain unusual situations such as a penicillin allergic patient with staphylococcal meningitis. If the CSF has not been sterilized within 48 hours, the administration of intrathecal vancomycin (20 mg) should be considered. Nephrotoxicity, ototoxicity, and phlebitis are adverse reactions of vancomycin.

Antifungal Agents

Therapy for fungal CNS infections has been limited for the most part to the use of amphotericin B.[35] Of the other available antifungal agents only 5-fluorocytosine (5-FC) and miconazole have been shown to be effective. Neither miconazole nor 5-FC, however, has replaced amphotericin B as the primary agent for serious fungal infections.[5,13,43,44]

Amphotericin B   is a polyene macrolide antibiotic which binds to cell membrane sterols. This binding results in increased cell permeability with membrane disruption and leakage of cytoplasmic contents. Amphotericin B must be given intravenously. Susceptible fungi, which include the majority of organisms which cause meningitis or brain abscess, are inhibited *in vitro* by 0.01 to 1.0 µg/ml of amphotericin B. *Aspergillus* species and Zygomycetes are, however, frequently resistant *in vitro*. The usual daily intravenous dose of 0.6 to 1.0 mg/kg results in serum levels of 0.5 to 2.0 µg/ml, thus exceeding the minimum fungistatic concentration (MFC) of most fungi. The CSF penetration of amphotericin B is poor and CSF levels are usually 2–10 percent of serum concentrations. Despite such poor CSF entry, intravenous amphotericin B is effective in immunologically intact patients with meningitis caused by most fungi except *Coccidiodes immitis*. Infection caused by this organism is the only definite indication for both intravenous and intrathecal amphotericin B therapy.[43]

There is no universal agreement as to the optimum daily dose, total dose or duration of amphotericin B therapy. What appears important in all regimens is prolonged treatment, in most instances for 6–12 weeks.[5] The *usual* total dose ranges between 1.5–3.0 g. With a non-emergent clinical situation, during the first week of therapy, the daily intravenous dose is increased gradually by 5–10 mg increments per day to a level of 0.6–1.0 mg/kg/day and kept there for one to two more weeks. This is then followed by therapy with 1–1.5 mg/kg/day every other day. The alternate day drug schedule has been shown to be effective and is less toxic. This regimen can then be used for the duration of the treatment. If the patient is seriously ill, an effective dosage level (0.6–1.0 mg/kg/day) can be reached more rapidly, within 24–36 hours, by following a 1 mg test-dose (given to all patients to exclude severe reactions) with 10–15 mg every 6 hours for the first day. Thereafter, an infusion of 40–60 mg (approximately 0.6 mg/kg) should be given once daily over the usual 6–8 hour interval. Alternate day therapy should not be used in immunosuppressed or severely ill patients until the infection is clearly under control.

The adverse effects of intravenous amphotericin B include azotemia (virtually always encountered), hypokalemia, hypomagnesemia, and anemia. Directly related to the infusion are phlebitis, fever, chills, nausea, vomiting, and headache. The infusion-related complications which tend to abate with continued therapy can be reduced by adding 1000 units of heparin (for phlebitis) and 15–20 mg hydrocortisone (for fever and chills) to the infusion bottle, and by pretreating the patient with bendryl (25–50 mg orally or intramuscularly), compazine (5–10 mg orally or intramuscularly), or aspirin. The dose of amphotericin B should be reduced or omitted for several days when the blood urea exceeds 50 mg percent. Blood-urea nitrogen and creatinine should be maintained under 50 mg percent and 3.5 mg percent, respectively.[5]

At present, intrathecal amphotericin B is indicated in only a few instances. When employed, intraventricular instillation is recommended through a subcutaneous reservoir such as an Ommaya reservoir rather than by intralumbar or intracisternal injection.[14] Lumbar administration of amphotericin B is associated with local pain, headache, and arachnoiditis or radiculitis, and cannot be used if a subarachnoid block is present. Although experience is limited, amphotericin B in a 10 percent glucose solution given by the lumbar route appears to result in fairly consistent delivery to the basal cisterns. Cisternal injection requires fluoroscopic control and neurosurgical skill, and is not without local complications.

Regardless of the route of intrathecal administration, the initial dose should be small (0.05–1.0 mg/day) and gradually increased over several days to 0.3–1.0 mg usually given 1–3 times per week. Intrathecal hydrocortisone (25 mg) may also be injected simultaneously to reduce irritative reactions. Once begun, intrathecal amphotericin B is usually continued until the patient has clearly responded to therapy, CSF cultures are negative, or serum and CSF serologic titers have decreased. In coccidioidal meningitis, intermittent intrathecal therapy is typically required for several years.[43]

5-fluorocytosine (5-FC), a synthetic fluorinated pyrimidine, exerts its chemotherapeutic effect by conversion within susceptible fungal cells to 5-fluorouracil, an antimetabolite. 5-FC has proved most useful in cryptococcal and Candida infections. It has also been shown to be effective *in vitro* against some Torulopsis and Aspergillus species.[5]

5-FC is well-absorbed orally and peak serum levels range between 50–100 μg/ml following a 4 g oral dose. It penetrates the CSF well and CSF levels are 50–80 percent of simultaneously determined serum concentrations. A major problem with 5-FC has been therapeutic failure associated with the development of organism resistance during therapy especially when suboptimal doses (i.e., less than the recommended 150 mg/kg/day) are used. Although cures have been reported in cryptococcal meningitis with 5-FC alone, few investigators suggest that this alone is the drug of choice for any of the fungal meningitides regardless of *in vitro* susceptibility. The relapse rate in patients with cryptococcal meningitis treated with 5-FC alone approximates 25 percent while with amphotericin B it is about 5–10 percent. Therapy with 5-FC alone should probably be reserved for certain patients who have relapsed after amphotericin B or for whom a strong contraindication to amphotericin B therapy is present. The promising role of combined 5-FC and amphotericin B therapy in cryptococcal meningitis is discussed below. The dosage of 5-FC must be reduced in renal failure. 5-FC side effects include skin rash, elevated transaminase levels, anemia, leukopenia, and thrombocytopenia.

Miconazole. This agent, a synthetic imidazole derivative, alters the permeability and respiratory metabolism of fungi.[13] Limited clinical experience with miconazole in coccidioidal meningitis and in a few cases of cryptococcal meningitis has been reported to be favorable. Miconazole, like 5-FC, should also be reserved for amphotericin B treatment failures or situations where amphotericin B is contraindicated since its role as a primary antifungal agent has not yet been clarified.

Miconazole is given intravenously in three divided doses for a total of 30 mg/kg/day for 4–8 weeks. Serum levels of 2–8 μg/ml result from a 10 mg/kg dose. Despite relatively poor CSF penetration, clinical responses have been observed with intravenous therapy alone. Miconazole can be safely administered intrathecally (20 mg daily or every second day) and this route should probably be used in addition to intravenous therapy in critically ill patients or in those failing to respond after a trial of parenteral therapy.[13]

Other Antifungal Agents

Iodides, 2-hydroxystilbamidine, and clotrimazole have no place in the treatment of fungal infections of the meninges or brain.[5]

Antituberculous Agents

Isoniazid (INH),   the mainstay of all antituberculous regimens is tuberculocidal, well-absorbed orally, and readily passes into the CSF regardless of the degree of meningeal inflammation. CSF levels of INH approximate 75–99 percent of serum concentrations.[2,35] Since resistance of tubercle bacilli to INH occurs throughout the world and especially in the Orient, all isolates should be tested for susceptibility. Suggested doses of INH range from 5–20 mg/kg/day. Initially, 10 mg/kg/day is sufficient for severely ill patients. The dose can be reduced to a 5 mg/kg (i.e., 300 mg/day for adults) after about 4–6 weeks. INH and one other drug should be continued for a total of 18–24 months.

Major adverse reactions to INH include hepatitis (more common in rapid acetylators) and peripheral neuropathy (more frequent in slow acetylators or in patients receiving high-dose INH). INH should be discontinued immediately in patients with hepatitis symptoms if elevated serum bilirubin or transaminase levels are present. Neuropathy is preventable and responds to pyridoxine (50–100 mg/day). Less common adverse reactions to INH include seizures, autonomic dysfunction, encephalopathy, optic neuritis, acute psychosis, fever, polyarthritis, a lupus-like illness, and a variety of hematologic abnormalities. Most of these respond promptly to discontinuation of INH.

Ethambutol   is tuberculostatic, well-absorbed orally, and peak blood levels of 4–5 μg/ml are achieved after single doses of 25 mg/kg. In the absence of meningeal inflammation, ethambutol does not pass into the CSF; however, CSF levels in patients with tuberculous meningitis vary from 15–50 percent of serum concentrations.[6] Most *M. tuberculosis* strains are inhibited by 1 μg/ml of ethambutol, a concentration readily obtained in CSF after a 25 mg/kg oral dose. High doses (25 mg/kg/day in adults) should be used for the first 6–8 weeks to assure adequate CSF levels; followed by a 15 mg/kg/day dose thereafter. Toxicity to ethambutol includes optic neuritis (which is an indication to reduce the dosage) and hyperuricemia.

Rifampin is an extremely effective, tuberculocidal agent which adequately enters the CSF in the presence of meningeal inflammation.[15] The drug, like ethambutol, is available only for oral administration. Most *M. tuberculosis* strains are inhibited by 0.5 μg/ml or less and primary resistance is rare. Single daily adult doses of 10 mg/kg (600 mg) result in serum levels ranging between 4–32 μg/ml; CSF levels approximate 20 percent of serum values. Hepatitis is the major adverse reaction to rifampin and there is some evidence to suggest that INH plus rifampin increases the risk of drug-induced hepatitis. Skin rash, gastrointestinal intolerance, hemolytic anemia, and thrombocytopenia may also occur.

Antiviral Agents

Vidarabine (adenine arabinoside, ARA-A), a purine nucleoside analog, has recently been shown in a controlled study to be effective in the treatment of *Herpes simplex* (Herpes hominis) encephalitis and represents a major advance in antiviral chemotherapy.[46] This agent may also be beneficial in some of the complications of disseminated varicella-zoster virus infections including encephalitis.

Vidarabine therapy, which should be used only after brain biopsy has confirmed the specific diagnosis, is given intravenously (15 mg/kg/day) over 12 hours in concentrations not exceeding 0.7 mg/ml of standard infusion solutions. Therapy must be initiated early in the course (i.e. before the onset of coma) to have a beneficial effect. At a dosage of 15 mg/kg/day, significant leukopenia or thrombocytopenia is infrequent.

MENINGITIS

General Considerations

Infection of the meninges initially causes inflammation and congestion of superficial cerebral arteries and veins. With exudation of inflammatory cells into the subarachnoid space and into the ventricular system, the sulci and basilar cisterns fill with exudate. The inflammatory response may cause obstruction of cerebrospinal fluid flow either due to involvement of the arachnoid granulations or aqueduct and lead to increased intracranial pressure. Thrombosis of large and small superficial arteries and veins leads to small foci of cerebral ischemia, cerebral edema, infarction, and abscess formation.

Successful treatment of patients with infectious meningitis depends not only upon appropriate antimicrobial therapy, but also upon many other factors including early recognition, accurate microbial identification, aggressive supportive care, surgical intervention when indicated, and management of related complications. Although this section will deal primarily with antimicrobial therapy, it is worth re-emphasizing several other aspects.

Probably most important for patients with meningitis is the prompt recognition that meningitis is present. Since, in some instances the presentation of microbial meningitis may be subtle with none of the typical signs or symptoms, a lumbar puncture (LP) should always be performed whenever the possibility of meningitis has been raised.

The importance of identifying the specific organism responsible for meningitis cannot be over-emphasized. While the identity of the causative organism has obvious therapeutic implications, other considerations regarding the particular organism involved include the pathogenesis of infection, public health measures, and prognosis. Careful attention must be directed toward obtaining smears and cultures of appropriate CSF specimens. Sites outside the CNS such as blood, wound drainage, sinus exudate or skin lesions should also be assiduously cultured to facilitate isolation of the pathogen. Serologic methods performed on either CSF or blood by counterimmunoelectrophoresis (CIE) or other techniques may also rapidly identify the responsible pathogen.

Also important in the successful management of patients with microbial meningitis is awareness of the potential complications, both neurologic and systemic, which may develop (or may already be present) and an understanding of how to manage these complications. Examples of complications are listed in Table 11-4 and include hyponatremia from inappropriate ADH secretion, aspiration pneumonia, disseminated intravascular coagulation, cerebral edema or abscess formation, subdural effusions, seizures, cortical vein thrombosis, persistence of parameningeal or distant foci of suppuration, and late hydrocephalus.[9,41] These complications emphasize, in turn, the necessity of identifying as clearly as possible the pathogenesis of the infection which led to meningitis. Identification of the mechanism by which infection gained access to the CNS depends on a high index of clinical suspicion and a knowledge of the various mechanisms by which meningitis may arise (Table 11-3). The importance of knowing how infection developed is related to potential changes in therapy which this knowledge may dictate. Such would be the case in a patient with meningitis with bacteremia from a distant pulmonary empyema or intraabdominal suppurative focus; with extension of infection from a contiguous process such as mastoiditis, otitis media, or cranial osteomyelitis, a dural leak, or endocarditis. If these lesions are present and appear to be responsible for meningitis, surgical intervention may be required in some instances, or prolonged parenteral antimicrobial therapy in others.

The major determinant of successful management is prompt and appropriate antimicrobial therapy. This is defined as treatment initiated immediately with an agent which adequately penetrates into the CSF and to which the organism causing meningitis is susceptible. The pharmacology of the commonly employed antimicrobial agents in central nervous system (CNS) infections as well as general considerations regarding their use has been dealt with in a previous section. Considered below are specific therapeutic regimens for patients with meningitis from two standpoints: first, situations in which the etiologic agent has been identified (Table 11-7); and second, situations in which the etiologic agent has not yet been identified (Tables 11-5 and 11-6). For this latter group, knowledge of specific predisposing factors such as the patient's age, evidence of contiguous infection or trauma coupled with the type of CSF response will, in most instances, permit the clinician to make an educated presumptive microbiologic diagnosis and to initiate adequate antimicrobial therapy. Tables 11-5 and 11-7 summarize these recommended treatment regimens.

Bacterial Meningitis

Infection Caused by Gram-Positive and Gram-Negative Cocci

Streptococcus pneumoniae and *Neisseria meningitidis* continue to be the most common bacteria causing pyogenic meningitis in immunologically intact persons over 14 years of age. The majority of patients with pneumococcal meningitis have readily identifiable sources of infection such as otitis media, mastoiditis, sinusitis, or pneumonia, but approximately 30 percent will have no apparent source of infection.[41] An upper respiratory source is presumably present with most meningococcal infections, but is not usually clinically evident.

Ten to fourteen days of high-dose intravenous penicillin G (Table 11-7) remains the regimen of choice for these two infections. Ampicillin is equally effective but is more costly and causes more adverse reactions than penicillin. For penicillin-allergic patients, parenteral chloramphenicol may be employed. Erythromycin is also adequate, though experience with this drug is limited. Since approximately 70 percent of *N. meningitidis* are resistant to sulfonamides, these agents should not be used as initial therapy. Intrathecal administration of penicillin is rarely warranted because adequate CSF levels are usually attained with intravenous therapy. Since 10–15 percent of pneumococci are resistant to tetracycline, this agent should not be used. Although effective against both *S. pneumoniae* and *N. meningitidis*, neither clindamycin nor the currently available cephalosporins (cephalothin, cephaloridine, cefazolin) should be used in treating any type of CNS infection because of unreliable penetration.

Non-pneumococcal streptococcal meningitis is rare in adults unless predisposing disorders are present, such as head trauma, neurosurgical procedures,

Table 11-5 / Antimcrobial Therapy of Presumed Meningitis of Unknown Etiology

Immune Status	Age	CSF Gram Stain	Likely Organisms	Antimicrobial Regimen of Choice	Daily Dose	Route of Administration	Alternative Regimen for Patients with Penicillin Allergy
Normal	Neonate (0–2 month)	Negative	*Escherichia coli* Group B Beta-Hemolytic streptococcus	Ampicillin and Gentamicin	75–150 mg/kg 5 mg/kg	IV IV	Chloramphenicol and Gentamicin
Normal	Children (2 months–15 years)	Negative	*Haemophilus influenza* *Streptococcus pneumoniae* *Neisseria meningitidis*	Chloramphenicol and Ampicillin	50–75 mg/kg 75–150 mg/kg	IV IV	
Normal	Adult	Negative	*Streptococcus pneumoniae* *Neisseria meningitidis*	Ampicillin	12 g	IV	Chloramphenicol
Altered	Adult	Negative	*Listeria monocytogenes* Gram-Negative bacilli *Streptococcus pneumoniae* *Neisseria meningitidis* *Cryptococcus neoformans*	Penicillin and Chloramphenicol and Gentamicin Amphotericin B*	24 million units 4–8 g 5 mg/kg 0.5 mg/kg	IV IV IV IV	Chloramphenicol and Gentamicin
Normal or Altered	Adult	Gram-Positive Cocci	*Streptococcus pneumoniae* Beta-hemolytic streptococcus *Staphylococcus aureus*	Nafcillin	12 g	IV	Vancomycin and Chloramphenicol
Normal or Altered	Adult	Gram-Negative Bacilli	*Escherichia coli* Klebsiella-Enterobacteriaceae *Pseudomonas aeruginosa*	Chloramphenicol and Gentamicin Gentamicin Carbenicillin	8 g 5 mg/kg 5–10 mg 0.5 g/kg	IV IV Intrathecal IV	Gentamicin (iv and IT) Chloramphenicol
Normal or Altered	Adult	Gram-Positive Bacilli	*Listeria monocytogenes* *Clostridia* species *Bacillus* species } indwelling Diphtheroids } prosthesis	Penicillin	24 million units	IV	Chloramphenicol
Normal or Altered	Adult	Gram-Negative Cocci	*Neisseria meningitidis* *Neisseria gonorrhoea*	Penicillin	24 million units	IV	Chloramphenicol

*Rarely indicated as initial therapy unless the patient is moribund or deteriorating on antibacterial regimen.

Table 11-6 / Antimicrobial Therapy of Presumed Brain Abscess of Unknown Etiology

Source of Infection	Immune Status	Likely Organisms	Antimicrobial Regimen of Choice	Daily Dose	Route	Alternative Antimicrobial Regimen for Penicillin Allergic Patient
None	Normal	Anaerobes Viridans streptococci Streptococcus pneumoniae	Chloramphenicol	4–8 g	IV	
None	Altered	Enterobacteriaceae Pseudemonas aeruginosa Anaerobes Aspergillus Mucormycosis Nocardia	Chloramphenicol and Gentamicin (Amphotericin B*) (Sulfa-Trimethoprim)	4–8 g 5 mg/kg 0.5 mg/kg	IV IV IV	
Sinus	Normal	Viridans streptococci Anaerobes Haemophilus influenza Streptococcus pneumoniae	Chloramphenicol	4–8 g	IV	
Middle ear or mastoid	Normal	Enterobacteriaceae Pseudomonas aeruginosa Staphylococcus aureus Anaerobes Streptococci	Nafcillin and Chloramphenicol and Gentamicin	12 g 4–8 g 5 mg/kg	IV IV IV	Vancomycin† and Chloramphenicol and Gentamicin
Neuro-surgery or Penetrating Trauma	Normal	Enterobacteriaceae Pseudomonas aeruginosa Staphylococcus aureus Anaerobes Streptococcus Group A	Nafcillin and Chloramphenicol and Gentamicin	12 g 4–8 g 5 mg/kg	IV IV IV	Vancomycin† and Chloramphenicol and Gentamicin

*If the patient is moribund or deteriorates on antibacterial therapy institution of Amphotericin B should be considered.
†Since not all staphylococci are sensitive to Chloramphenicol, Vancomycin should be used until the sensitivity to Chloramphenicol is established.

malignancy, or subacute bacterial endocarditis. In neonates and infants, however, Group B beta-hemolytic streptococci are a common cause of meningitis. For all streptococcal meningitides except those caused by Group D streptococci, high dose intravenous penicillin is the drug of choice. Chloramphenicol is the alternative in patients who are allergic to penicillin. For the patients with Group D streptococcal (enterococcal, *S. faecalis*) meningitis (a rare occurrence), penicillin alone is not effective and ampicillin is the drug of choice.[3] For patients with Group D streptococcal meningitis who fail to respond to ampicillin alone, a parenterally administered aminoglycoside should be added. Should improvement not occur, intrathecal aminoglycoside treatment (vide infra) should be started. Intravenous vancomycin can be used in patients with enterococcal meningitis who are allergic to penicillin.

Staphylococcal Meningitis. Meningitis caused by *S. aureus* is very unusual in the absence of specific preceding disorder such as head trauma, neurosurgery, invasive diagnostic studies (i.e., myelography), head and neck tumors, or acute bacterial endocarditis.[9,41] *S. epidermidis* (coagulase negative) infections may also follow head injury or craniotomy, but typically occur in the presence of indwelling foreign bodies such as ventricular shunts or reservoirs.[38] Pending sensitivity testing, a penicillinase (beta-lactamase) · resistant semisynthetic penicillin should be employed initially in staphylococcal infections since resistance to penicillin, even among community-acquired strains, is frequent. Nafcillin, methicillin, and oxacillin all readily enter the CSF. Nafcillin is preferred because it is 3–7 times more active against *S. aureus* than oxacillin or methicillin and it appears to cause fewer adverse reactions than does methicillin. Since methicillin-resistant staphylococci pose a problem in some hospitals, sensitivity testing should always be performed. Vancomycin is effective against most methicillin-resistant *S. aureus* strains. Similarly, since *S. epidermidis* isolates tend to vary in their susceptibility to commonly used antistaphylococcal agents, every CSF or blood isolate should be tested for sensitivity.

Patients with staphylococcal meningitis who are allergic to penicillin pose a special problem. Parenteral clindamycin or cephalosporins cannot be used since they penetrate CSF poorly. Chloramphenicol and erythromycin are effective against many, but not all staphylococci; hence, their use as initial therapy is hazardous. Vancomycin penetrates into CSF adequately, is bactericidal against almost all staphylococci, and has been effective in limited clinical experience.[20] Thus, vancomycin is probably the best alternative for patients with penicillin allergy until the susceptibility of the organism is known.

Intrathecal vancomycin (20 mg/day) may also be added if CSF cultures remain positive after 48 hours. Intrathecal cephaloridine (10–50 mg/day) plus intravenous cephalothin has also been suggested for patients in whom the penicillin "allergy" is not of the potentially cross-reacting anaphylactoid type. Rapid

Table 11-7 / Antimicrobial Therapy for Central Nervous System Infection of Known Etiology

Causative Organisms	Antimicrobial Regimen of Choice*	Daily Dose	Route of Administration	Antimicrobial Regimen for Pencillin Allergic Patients
A. Bacteria				
Actinomyces israelii	Penicillin	24 million units	IV	Erythromycin
Clostridia species	Penicillin	24 million units	IV	Chloramphenicol
Escherichia coli	Chloramphenicol**	4–8 g	IV	
Francisella tularensis	Chloramphenicol	4–8 g	IV	
Haemophilus influenzae	Chloramphenicol and	4–8 g	IV	
	Ampicilin	12g	IV	
Klebsiella pneumoniae	Chloramphenicol**	4-8g	IV	
Listeria monocytogenes	Ampicillin	12 g	IV	Chloramphenicol
Mycobacterium tuberculosis	Isoniazid and	300 mg	po or IV	
	Ethambutal and	15–25 mg/kg	po	
	Rifampin	600 mg	po	
Mycoplasma pneumoniae	Erythromycin	2 g	IV	
Neisseria gonorrhoeae	Penicillin	24 million units	IV	Erythromycin
Neisseria meningitidis	Penicillin	24 million units	IV	Chloramphenicol
Nocardia species	Trimethoprim and	1200–1600 mg	po	
	Sulfamethoxazole	6–9 g	po	
Proteus species	Ampicillin**	12 g	IV	Gentamicin
Pseudemonas aeruginosa	Gentamicin† and Gentamicin	5 mg/kg 5–10 mg	IV Intrathecal	Gentamicin alone
	Carbinicillin	0.5 g/kg	IV	
Salmonella species	Chloramphenicol	4–8 g	IV	
Serrata species	Gentamicin**	5 mg/kg	IV	
	Gentamicin†	5–10 mg	Intrathecal	
Staphylococcus aureus	Nafcillin	12 g	IV	Vancomycin†
Staphylococcus epidermidis	Vancomycin	2 g	IV	
Streptococci				
Viridans	Penicillin	24 million units	IV	Chloramphenicol

B hemolytic	Penicillin	24 million units	IV	Chloramphenicol
Group D	Ampicillin	24 million units	IV	Vancomycin
pneumoniae	Penicillin	24 million units	IV	Chloramphenicol
Anaerobes	Chloramphenicol	4–8 g	IV	
B. Fungi				
Blastomyces dermatidis	Amphotericin B	0.5 mg/kg	IV	
Candida albicans	Amphotericin B	0.5 mg/kg	IV	
Coccidioides immitis	Amphotericin B and	0.5 mg/kg	IV	
	Amphotericin B	0.5–1 mg	Intrathecal	
Cryptococcus neoformans	Amphotericin B and	0.5 mg/kg	IV	
	5 Fluorocytosine	150–200 mg/kg	po	
Histoplasma capsulatrum	Amphotericin B	0.5 mg/kg	IV	
Sporotrichum schenckii	Amphotericin B	0.5 mg/kg	IV	
C. Rickettsia				
Rickettsia species	Chloramphenicol	4–8 g	IV	
D. Spirochetes				
Borrelia species	Chloramphenicol	4–8 g	IV	
Leptospira interrogans	Penicillin	24 million units	IV	Tetracycline
Treponema pallidum	Penicillin	24 million units	IV	Erythromycin
E. Protozoa				
Endameoba histolytica	Metronidazole	2250 mg	po	
Naeglaria	Amphotericin B	0.5 mg/kg	IV	
Plasmodium falciparum	Quinine	up to 1950 mg	po or IV	
Toxoplasma gondii	Sulfadiazine and	4 g	IV	
	Pyrimethamine	75 mg (day 1)	po	
F. Flagellates				
Trypanosoma gambiensis	Suramin and	1 g		
	Melarsoprol	2–3.6 mg/kg	IV	
Trypanosoma rhodesiensis	Suramin and	1 g	IV	
	Melarsopol	2–3.6 mg/kg	IV	

*The antimicrobial regimen of choice has been selected on the basis of the penetration of the drug into the CNS, the likely sensitivity of the specific microorganism, and published experience with regard to clinical response. In every case the sensitivity of each pathogen should be measured by a quantitative method.

**Enterobacteriaceae (e.g., *E. Coli*, *Klebsiella* species, *Enterobacter* species), *Proteus* species, and *Serratia* species can occasionally be resistant to the drug of choice listed. If the sensitivity of the organism is in doubt, an aminoglycoside should be administered by intravenous route (and intrathecal route when applicable), in addition to the drug of choice until the sensitivity is established.

†For meningitis, intrathecal gentamicin should be administered in addition to systemic antibiotic.

‡Since not all staphylococci are sensitive to chloramphenicol, Vancomycin should be used until the sensitivity of the staphylococcus to chloramphenicol is established.

desensitization to a penicillinase-resistant penicillin may also be attempted. Probably most prudent is the use of intravenous vancomycin until sensitivity testing suggests a less toxic agent whose CSF penetration is well-documented such as chloramphenicol. Because of limited experience with vancomyin, patients who receive this agent should have a repeat LP within the first 24–48 hours of therapy to monitor CSF culture, CSF vancomycin levels and CSF bactericidal activity.

Parenteral antistaphylococcal therapy should be continued for a minimum of 14 days. If there is a parameningeal focus of infection (i.e. infected foreign body, bone, devitalized tissue, hematoma) prompt surgical intervention is necessary if a favorable clinical outcome is to be attained. Patients with underlying *S. aureus* endocarditis require 4–6 weeks of intravenous therapy. Treatment of CSF shunt and reservoir infections will be considered separately.

Meningitis caused by other gram-positive or gram-negative cocci such as gonococci (*N. gonorrhoeae*) and anaerobic cocci (peptostreptococcus, peptococcus) is exceedingly rare. Penicillin therapy is usually adequate.[28]

When faced with a patient with purulent meningitis where gram-positive cocci are found on CSF smear, but where the Quellung reaction (diagnostic for pneumococci) and the CIE test (for pneumococcal antigen) are both negative, high-dose nafcillin therapy should be initiated in order to include coverage of the rare case of staphylococcal meningitis. Nafcillin provides adequate coverage for *S. aureus* as well as *S. pneumoniae* and other streptococci. If the Quellung reaction is positive or if culture results subsequently indicate a penicillin sensitive infection, the therapy should then be changed to penicillin alone.

Infection Caused by Gram-Positive Bacilli

This group of organisms includes *Listeria monocytogenes*, *Clostridium* species, *Bacillus* species and diptheroids. Infection caused by *Bacillus* and diptheroid species rarely occur except in patients with an indwelling CNS prosthesis (see CSF shunt infections).

Clostridial meningitis is rare and is usually a postoperative complication or is associated with brain abscess. Both penicillin and chloramphenicol are effective against *Clostridium* species.[41]

Listeria monocytogenes infection is a relatively common cause of meningitis in immunocompromised patients such as renal transplant recipients and those with solid or hematopoietic malignancies.[10] Listeria meningitis may also occur in immunologically intact patients of any age. Good clinical results have been obtained in patients with Listeria meningitis treated with penicillin or ampicillin. Treatment failures, however, have been reported with both agents, presumably because (in contrast to their action against most gram-positive organisms), penicillin and ampicillin appear to be only bacteriostatic against *L.*

monocytogenes. Nevertheless, they remain the drugs of choice. Chloramphenicol or erythromycin may be used for patients with penicillin allergy. Enhanced *in vitro* killing of *L. monocytogenes* has been demonstrated with penicillin or ampicillin plus an aminoglycoside. For patients who respond poorly to a single agent, combination therapy could be considered.

Infection Caused by Gram-Negative Bacilli

There are numerous gram-negative bacilli which can cause meningitis in patients of each age category. Treatment regimens for gram-negative bacillary meningitis are complicated by the resistance of some gram-negative bacilli to all antibiotics which penetrate the meninges well. Initial treatment regimens must be formulated on the likelihood that such a resistant organism is the causative agent. In neonates, *E. coli* is a common cause of meningitis, while *Pseudomonas* species are unusual. Thus, intravenous ampicillin and kanamycin have traditionally been the initial regimen of choice, and intrathecal aminoglycoside has not been considered necessary.[28] (If intravenous aminoglycoside is to be used as part of the initial regimen, poor penetration of the meninges notwithstanding, gentamicin or tobramycin should be used instead of kanamycin due to greater safety and the growing number of kanamycin resistant but gentamicin or tobramycin sensitive *E. coli* in nurseries). If the isolate is sensitive to ampicillin, the aminoglycoside should be discontinued. However, if the organism is sensitive only to an aminoglycoside, then intrathecal treatment must be considered because of the poor CSF penetration of all the aminoglycosides. Small amounts of systemically administered gentamicin, tobramycin, and kanamycin pass inflamed meninges, and cures without intrathecal injections do occur. Since mortality for gram-negative bacillary neonatal meningitis (about 30 percent) has not yet been shown to be reduced by initial intrathecal therapy, one is justified in using intravenous therapy while awaiting either repeatedly positive CSF cultures (suggestive of ventriculitis) or clinical deterioration before adding intrathecal drug.[18] Initial intrathecal therapy is usually given by the lumbar route, and intraventricular adminstration may ultimately be necessary.[23,24]

Haemophilus influenzae is the most common cause of bacterial meningitis in infants older than two months and in children under the age of 14 years.[39] It is less frequent after the age of 5 and rare in normal adults. Parenteral ampicillin or chloramphenicol have been the antibiotics of choice for this infection in both children and adults. Ampicillin-resistant *H. influenzae* (almost always Type B) are being encountered more frequently and there have been scattered reports of treatment failure with ampicillin despite the presence of a sensitive organism. Chloramphenicol resistant *H. influenzae* bacilli have been reported, but are still rare. No organisms have been resistant to both ampicillin and chloramphenicol. Prudent initial antimicrobial therapy for suspected or proved *H. influenzae* meningitis should include both ampicillin and chloramphenicol until the sensitivity of the causative organism is known.

Other than that caused by *H. influenzae,* meningitis in children caused by gram-negative bacilli is unusual except when certain well-defined predisposing factors are present (Table 11-3). The same factors are typically found in adults with gram-negative bacillary infections, and *E. coli, Pseudomonas aeruginosa,* and Klebsiella are most frequently causative organisms, while meningitis caused by species of Serratia, Proteus, Enterobacter, Salmonella, and anaerobic bacilli occur on rare occasions.

The most reliable initial antibiotic regimen for gram-negative bacillary meningitis is intravenous chloramphenicol plus the combination of parenteral and intralumbar aminoglycoside therapy using either gentamicin or tobramycin. If Pseudomonas is suspected, intravenous carbenicillin should be employed in the initial regimen. Chloramphenicol is highly effective in meningitis caused by susceptible organisms and carbenicillin may prove to be effective, but neither agent (nor ampicillin) can be recommended as initial therapy alone because so many gram-negative bacilli are resistant to them. Should the isolated bacteria subsequently prove sensitive to chloramphenicol or ampicillin, then high-dose intravenous regimen (in adults, chloramphenicol 6–8 g/day; ampicillin 8–12 g/day) can be used and the aminoglycoside discontinued. Resistance to chloramphenicol developing during therapy has been recently reported in patients with gram-negative bacillary meningitis. Thus, when this agent is used alone, one must follow CSF cultures carefully. Because of the effectiveness and broad spectrum of gentamicin and tobramycin, kanamycin and polymyxin B no longer have a role in the treatment of gram-negative bacillary meningitis. The spectrum of these latter two drugs' activity is limited, they are relatively more toxic, and the efficacy of polymyxin B is dubious.

If the causative agent is not sensitive to an antibiotic which penetrates the meninges well, intrathecal aminoglycoside therapy is necessary. Rarely are gram-negative bacilli resistant to gentamicin or tobramycin. Since intravenous aminoglycoside does not penetrate the meninges well, intralumbar aminoglycoside therapy should be administered as soon as gram-negative bacilli are implicated.[23,33,34] Intralumbar aminoglycoside therapy often results in suboptimal ventricular fluid levels, but this route of administration is usually chosen initially because it is minimally invasive and often results in clinical improvement. However, for patients who appear moribund on admission, respond poorly to treatment, or relapse, an intraventricular reservoir (such as an Ommaya reservoir) should be inserted, and the aminoglycoside administered directly into the ventricles.[23]

In rare instances, the gram-negative bacilli may be resistant to gentamicin and tobramycin. A few of these resistant organisms will be sensitive to amikacin, another aminoglycoside. In most cases, urgent consultation with an experienced referral center will be necessary in order to assess by *in vitro* studies possible synergistic combinations. Prognosis for meningitis caused by these resistant organisms is extremely poor.

Gram-negative bacillary meningitis caused by anaerobes such as Bacteroides or fusobacterial species is unusual but may be associated with brain abscess, head trauma, and neurosurgical procedures. Aminoglycosides are not effective against anaerobes. Chloramphenicol is appropriate therapy, particularly for *B. fragilis*. Penicillin, ampicillin or carbenicillin can be used if the organism is sensitive to them.

Infection Caused by Multiple Organisms

Polymicrobial bacterial meningitis occurs infrequently, and has been observed most often in infants or adults with underlying CNS diseases, anatomic defects, or ventricular shunts. *H. influenzae* is the single most common isolate, followed in frequency by *N. meningitidis, S. pneumoniae,* and *E. coli.*[41] The initial regimen must be chosen on the basis of the predisposing lesion and the CSF gram stain, and should have a broad spectrum. Chloramphenicol is a logical therapeutic choice pending culture results.

Infection of Cerebrospinal Shunts or Reservoirs

Cerebrospinal fluid shunts and reservoirs sometimes become infected. Infection usually presents within 1–2 months of insertion or can be related to a transient bacteremia or prosthesis manipulation.[14,38] *S. epidermidis* is the most common organism responsible for infection in indwelling CSF appliances such as ventriculosystemic shunts, ventriculostomy tubes, and subcutaneous reservoirs of the Ommaya type. Shunt or reservoir infections may be caused by other indolent pathogens such as bacillus and diphtheroid species. *S. aureus* and gram-negative enteric bacilli may cause infection of ventriculo-atrial shunts or ventriculo-ureteral or lumbar-ureteral shunts, respectively. Prophylactic antibiotics given in the perioperative period have not been shown to consistently reduce the incidence of bacterial infections of shunts. Fungal infection of indwelling CSF appliances has fortunately not been a common problem thus far although several cases of Candida shunt infections have been reported. The pathogenesis of shunt infections is not clear but since most episodes occur within 1–2 months of operation and the commonly involved organisms are part of the normal skin flora, colonization at the time of insertion (or subsequent manipulation) is likely.

There is no general agreement about the optimum therapy of shunt infections. The clinical spectrum of prosthesis infections varies from asymptomatic colonization to full-blown bacterial meningitis. Cures have been reported to occur spontaneously (rare), with antibiotic therapy alone (prolonged intravenous plus oral drug courses with or without local instillation), or with shunt removal or revision (with and without antibiotics). For infections in ventriculo-systemic shunts it is most prudent to combine removal of the entire shunt apparatus with a 10–14 day course of a parenteral antibiotic, as many cases are associated with bacteremia.[38] Another shunt can be inserted in a different anatomic location, preferably after 7–10 days of therapy, which presumably will have eradicated organisms remaining in the CSF. If reasons to keep the infected shunt in place are compelling, a prolonged trial of high-dose parenteral (one month) plus oral (1–2 months more) antimicrobial therapy may be combined with daily drug instillation into the shunt for 2–4 weeks.

Antibiotic levels and bactericidal activity should be measured in the shunt CSF as a guide to the adequacy of therapy. If relapse occurs, the shunt or reservoir must be removed if the infection is to be cured. Limited experience with Ommaya reservoir infections suggests that prolonged antimicrobial therapy can result in successful eradication without having to remove the reservoir. The choice of antibiotics is dictated by the organism isolated and its in vitro sensitivities: typically nafcillin or vancomycin for *S. epidermidis* or *S. aureus*, chloramphenicol or gentamicin for Bacillus species, penicillin or vancomycin for diptheroids, and gentamicin for gram-negative bacilli.

Infection Caused by Spirochaetales (Leptospirosis, Relapsing Fever, Rat Bite Fever, Syphilis)

Leptospirosis may be associated with meningitis, meningoencephalitis, or an asymptomatic sterile CSF pleocytosis. If initiated early (before the fourth or fifth day of illness), penicillin G or tetracycline may ameliorate the course of leptospirosis.

"Relapsing Fever" caused by a variety of *Borrelia* species may be associated with symptoms of meningitis or other cerebral manifestations. Treatment with chloramphenicol or tetracycline is effective in eliminating the infection.

Rate Bite Fever is caused by *Spirillum minus* or *Streptobacillus moniliformis* and can be associated with cranial nerve dysfunction, encephalitis and coma. Penicillin or tetracycline is effective for curing the infection.

CNS infection caused by *T. pallidum* may result in a variety of syndromes including syphilitic meningitis, meningovascular syphilis, paretic neurosyphilis (general paresis), tabes dorsalis, and optic atrophy. Penicillin G remains the drug of choice for all forms of syphylitic CNS infections: it is adequately spirocheticidal in concentrations exceeding 0.03 μg/ml. Presently recommended standard treatment regimens include intramuscular procaine penicillin G 1.2 million units given every other day for a total of 6–9 million units or intramuscular penicillin G benzathine 2.4 million units given once weekly for 3–4 weeks. Other regimens suggest procaine penicillin G 1.2 million units/day for 10–15 days. Treatment is most effective in asymptomatic (i.e., positive CSF serology only) or early symptomatic syphilis (meningitis, or meningovascular). Penicillin is moderately effective in early general paresis but usually is of no benefit in tabes dorsalis. Retreatment is indicated if clinical deterioration occurs or when persistent CSF pleocytosis and rising CSF serologic titers develop despite therapy.

Oral erythromycin and tetracycline (total dose 60 g) may be used in patients allergic to penicillin, though the efficacy of these regimens has not yet been extensively evaluated.

Persistence of *T. pallidum* in the CSF of some patients who have received the standard regimens for neurosyphilis has recently been reported.[42] Following benzathine penicillin G therapy for neurosyphilis,[30] CSF penicillin levels have been found to be highly variable (not detectable in 12 of 13 patients in one study). Both findings suggest the need to re-evaluate the currently recommended dosages of penicillin for neurosyphilis with strong consideration for high-dose (i.e., 10–20 million units/day) and a prolonged (i.e., 10 days) regimen of intravenous penicillin.

Viral Meningitis

Viral meningitis is usually a benign and self-limited infection. No specific therapy is available. It is important to emphasize that a variety of disorders, both infectious and non-infectious, may present with an aseptic meningitis syndrome and cause diagnostic confusion. Examples include cases of partially treated bacterial meningitis, leptospirosis, syphilis, tuberculous meningitis, certain parasitic infections, connective tissue diseases (e.g., systemic lupus erythematosus), subacute bacterial endocarditis, sarcoidosis, and mycoplasmal or rickettsial infections. Currently there is no effective antiviral agent for any type of viral meningitis.

Tuberculous Meningitis

For the treatment of tuberculous meningitis there are a number of effective antituberculous agents available which readily cross into the CSF.[2,6,15,35] Most patients with tuberculous meningitis have miliary infection. Isoniazid (INH) is the most important therapeutic agent as it has high activity, low toxicity, and excellent CSF penetration. Rifampin, ethambutol, ethionamide, and cycloserine also pass into the CSF well. Streptomycin penetrates variably depending upon the degree of meningeal inflammation.

Patients with tuberculous meningitis respond favorably to a variety of multi-drug regimens, most commonly those employing three agents simultaneously. Although the incidence of resistance of *M. tuberculosis* strains to INH is increasing in certain areas (especially the Far East), INH resistance is usually not a clinical problem since two other additional antituberculous agents, to which the organisms are almost always sensitive, are usually used initially. A combination of INH, rifampin, and ethambutol for 6–8 weeks and then INH plus ethambutol for the remainder of a two-year course is the program of choice. Ethambutol is preferable to rifampin for the long term because of rifampin's expense and its apparent potential for additive hepatotoxicity when used with INH. Either INH and rifampin or INH and ethambutol can be used without a third drug in less severe cases, but the seriousness of tuberculous meningitis usually indicates the need for a maximally effective, triple-drug regimen for the first two or three months. Streptomycin is still commonly used as a third drug, but the ease of administering orally effective drugs makes this agent less desirable. If the patient is unable to take medication by mouth, however, INH and streptomycin are the only agents available in parenteral form. There is no longer a role for intrathecal streptomycin. Meningitis caused by atypical mycobacteria is rare. These organisms vary widely in their susceptibility to the agents effective against *M. tuberculosis.* Initial therapy should include at least three of the major antimycobacterial drugs such as INH, ethambutal and rifampin.

The role of corticosteroid therapy in tuberculous meningitis remains controversial.[35] Although some studies have reported clinical improvement and earlier resolution of CSF abnormalities with the use of corticosteroids in tuberculous meningitis, mortality has not been shown to improve. Cerebral edema and CSF block, however, continue to be indications for steroid therapy.

Fungal Meningitis

CNS infections caused by fungi are not common, but most of the pathogenic fungi are capable of producing meningitis in adults or children given the right clinical settings.[5,10,13,31,35,43,44] Previously healthy, immunologically competent individuals may develop meningitis associated with disseminated coccidioidomycosis, histoplasmosis, sporotrichosis, and North and South American blastomycosis. With the exception of coccidioidomycosis, however, meningitis due to these other fungi is very unusual. Meningitis from these infections typically results from hematogenous dissemination from a primary pulmonary focus.

Meningitis caused by species of Candida, Aspergillus, Torulopsis, Phycomycetes (i.e., Mucor), and Cryptococcus is typically associated with primary immunologic or granulocytic abnormalities resulting from an underlying debilitating disorder (i.e., solid or hematologic neoplasms, and renal transplantation);

or the effects of drugs such as corticosteroids or cytotoxic agents.[10] Although an initial pulmonary focus is often present with these opportunistic infections, spread to the meninges from contiguous sites such as the paranasal sinuses, orbit, or brain abscess occurs. Approximately 50 percent of patients with cryptococcal meningitis are not immunosuppressed and have no apparent predisposition to infection. As previously noted, Candida species may also infect ventricular shunts.

Intravenous amphotericin B is the drug of choice for fungal meningitis.[5] This continues to be the case despite poor passage of the agent into the CSF (<10 percent of serum levels) because of the proven therapeutic efficacy of amphotericin B. Experience in treating meningeal infections with 5-fluorocytosine (5-FC) and miconazole has been limited. The usefulness of 5-FC alone is compromised by its narrow spectrum of antifungal activity and by the frequent emergence of resistance during treatment especially when used in submaximal doses. Cures have been reported, however, with the use of 5-FC alone in meningitis caused by sensitive organisms, and if amphotericin B cannot be given, prolonged treatment with 5-FC may be successful. Miconazole can be given intrathecally as well as intravenously. This drug may prove to be a useful alternative to amphotericin B for sensitive organisms, particularly for coccidioidomycosis.

What constitutes optimal amphotericin B therapy has not been clearly defined for any of the fungal meningidities with perhaps the exception of cryptococcal meningitis.[44] Prolonged amphotericin B therapy in all cases of fungal infection, however, is important, and 1.5 to 3 g of intravenous amphotericin B is generally given over 6–12 weeks. Approximately 75 percent of patients with cryptococcal meningitis respond to this regimen. In many instances, infection due to the opportunistic fungi (Candida, Aspergillus, Mucor), progresses rapidly before a significant amount of drug can be given.

The indications for intrathecal amphotericin B (usually delivered intraventricularly through a reservoir or injected intracisternally) are quite limited.[5] Coccidioidal meningitis is the one definite indication. In coccidioidal meningitis, intrathecal therapy is invariably necessary and often must be given intermittently for prolonged periods (years) long after the usual adjunctive course of intravenous amphotericin B (1–2 g) has been completed. Because of the high frequency of relapse in coccidioidal meningitis despite prolonged therapy with amphotericin B with or without subsequent miconazole, the terms "remission" or "suppression" of infection should probably be used rather than "cure". For no other fungal meningitis should intrathecal therapy be chosen as an initial regimen, unless the patient is desperately ill. If clinical deterioration occurs during intravenous therapy or repeated relapses occur, then intrathecal therapy may be indicated.

The treatment of cryptococcal infection deserves special mention because it is the most frequent cause of fungal meningitis in immunosuppressed patients. It is also the only fungal infection in which combination therapy (amphotericin B plus 5-FC) has been evaluated clinically. Recently, a regimen consisting of low-dose intravenous amphotericin B (20 mg/day) plus full-dose oral 5-FC (150–200 mg/kg/day) given daily for six weeks has appeared to be safe and efficacious.[44] This regimen may reduce the incidence of toxicity resulting from high-dose prolonged amphotericin B therapy and shorten the hospital stay. Emerging resistance to 5-FC during therapy does not appear to be a problem with the combination therapy. The usefulness of combination therapy in other fungal meningitides has not yet been demonstrated.

Meningitis Caused by Nocardia Asteroides and Actinomyces Israelii

Meningitis caused by these agents (considered by some to be fungi) is rare. Nocardiosis typically occurs in the setting of a debilitating underlying disease and the sulfonamides remain the recommended treatment. Actinomycosis is not usually associated with predisposing disorders. Spread to the meninges occurs from contiguous infection (jaw, cervical region, sinuses) and less often by hematogenous spread from thoracoabdominal source. Penicillin is the drug of choice for actinomycosis.

Parasitic Meningitis

A variety of both protozoan and helminthic infections may involve the CNS. Most often, there is a prominent encephalitic component to the meningeal syndrome.

Infection Caused by Protozoa

Malaria, amebiasis, trypanosomiasis, and toxoplasmosis are the protozoan infections common enough to warrant discussion.

Cerebral malaria is most frequently associated with *Plasmodium falciparum* infection. Because cerebral malaria requires urgent treatment and because chloroquine resistance is a substantial concern in many geographic locations, quinine is the drug of choice. The dose of quinine is 650 mg orally every 8 hours for 7–10 days. Quinine dihydrochloride (600 mg) can be given intravenously if oral medication cannot be taken. Chloroquine therapy is also efficacious, but should be used only if the physician knows with certainty that chloroquine resistance does not exist in the region where the malaria was acquired.

Intestinal amebae (*Entamoeba histolytica*) and the free-living soil and water amebae of the Acanthameba-Naegleria group may rarely cause meningoencephalitis. In *E. histolytica* infection, agents such as emetine and chlorquine have been used. Metronidazole, effective in both intestinal and hepatic amebiasis is probably effective, but has not been fully evaluated in CNS amebic infections. Most cases of Naegleria meningitis are rapidly fatal; but amphotericin B has proved useful in isolated instances.

Encephalitis may be associated with each of the three forms of trypanosomiasis. The African form responds to the suramin and melarsoprol.

There is little evidence that treatment alters the course or reverses the deficits of congenitially-acquired toxoplasmosis. CNS toxoplasmosis in the adult is most often associated with an underlying immunologic abnormality. The clinical syndrome is similar to that of a brain abscess. Pyrimethamine plus a sulfamonide regimen is the therapy of choice. Trimethoprim-sulfamethoxazole would be a logical alternative.

Infection Caused by Helminths

Helminthic infections may also infrequently involve the CNS, resulting in either meningitis (usually aseptic), meningoencephalitis, or a mass lesion. Therapy includes antimonials or niridazole (schistosomiasis), thiabendazole (trichinosis, strongyloidiasis), bithionol (paragonomiasis), and surgery (cystercercosis).

Infection Caused by M. pneumoniae, Chlamydia, and Rickettsiae

Aseptic meningitis and encephalitis may be associated with *Mycoplasma pneumoniae* infection, chlamydial (psittacosis) infections, or rickettsial infections (Rocky Mountain spotted fever, typhus and others). *M. pneumoniae* infection responds to either erythromycin or tetracycline. The latter agent is effective against psittacosis and rickettsial diseases. There is little evidence that these antimicrobials alter the course of the CNS manifestations. The pathogenesis of meningitis or meningoencephalitis associated with infection caused by these organisms has not yet been established. Thus, therapy is given for treatment of the pulmonary infection (*M. pneumoniae*, psittacosis, Q fever) or systemic rickettsial disease, and not specifically for the infrequently observed CNS manifestations.

Antimicrobial Therapy When Microbial Meningitis Is Suspected But Not Immediately Documented

In patients with signs, symptoms, and CSF abnormalities compatible with meningitis, a specific etiologic agent often cannot be identified using rapid diagnostic methods such as CSF Gram's stain, smear for acid-fast bacilli (AFB), India ink preparation, or counterimmunoelectrophoresis. Such patients include those with viral meningitis and 25 percent of patients with bacterial meningitis as well as patients with non-infectious syndromes such as carcinomatous meningitis and sarcoidosis. Since bacterial meningitis can be so rapidly destructive, broad-spectrum antibacterial therapy must be instituted until the etiology of the meningitis can be unequivocally established by culture, cytology, antibody test, or other diagnostic means. Considerations for initiating appropriate therapy differ depending on whether the patient is immunologically normal, immunologically altered, or has received antibiotic therapy prior to lumbar puncture.

Immunologically Normal Patients

Presumptive antibiotic therapy for immunologically normal patients with clinical signs of meningitis should be determined on the basis of the most likely causative organism for the patient's age group. When faced with an otherwise healthy, immunocompetent adult who is older than 15 years with purulent meningitis of unknown etiology, infection caused by *S. pneumoniae* or *N. meningitidis* is the most likely. Spontaneous meningitis caused by *S. aureus*, gram-negative bacilli, parasites, or fungi is rare in these patients. High-dose intravenous therapy with ampicillin or penicillin G is appropriate. Chloramphenicol should be substituted for patients with penicillin allergy. Some experts prefer chloramphenicol as initial therapy in this situation because of this drug's activity against *H. influenzae* despite the rarity of *H. influenzae* meningitis after the age of 15 in otherwise healthy individuals. There is no advantage in using several of these drugs together and chloramphenicol may actually antagonize the action of penicillin or ampicillin because of its bacteriostatic action. We prefer ampicillin (12 g/day) in this setting.

In an otherwise healthy neonate or infant (with no congenital CNS or cranial defect), parenteral ampicillin plus gentamicin is the regimen of choice for purulent meningitis of unknown etiology. This regimen is effective against 90–95 percent of the bacteria isolated from infants in the 1–30 day and 30–60 day old age groups. Intrathecal aminoglycoside therapy should be considered early if the infant is moribund, if the clinical deterioration ensues, or if CSF cultures remain positive.[18] For healthy children from 2 months to 14 years of age, chloramphenicol and ampicillin are adequate initial therapy.

Fungal meningitis rarely occurs in immunologically normal patients, but cryptococcosis and coccidioidomycosis must be considered. In immunocompetent hosts, cryptococcal meningitis is not usually a rapidly progressive disease. Therapy with amphotericin B can therefore be withheld until cultures, serology, or an India ink preparation indicate this diagnosis. Coccidioidal meningitis should be suspected in an endemic area, but as in cryptococcal disease, meningitis is often not fulminant, and presumptive therapy can uusally be withheld until the diagnosis is proven. Tuberculous meningitis usually presents as a subacute or chronic process, but can present acutely. In the absence of AFB on smear of the CSF, antituberculous therapy should be initiated if there is evidence suggesting mycobacterial disease elsewhere (e.g., cavitary lung lesion), if there is neurological deterioration despite antibacterial therapy, or if the patient is extremely ill.

It is important to remember that viral meningitis may closely mimic bacterial meningitis both clinically and in CSF findings. In viral infections CSF white cell counts can be as high as 1000–2000/mm³ (with 90–100 percent polymorphonuclear leucocytes), protein may be elevated to 150 mg percent, and CSF sugar may be as low as 35–40 mg percent. If a viral infection is strongly suspected on the basis of history and physical findings, it is justified to withhold therapy for 6–8 hours and to repeat the lumbar puncture if (1) a careful Gram's stain of centrifuged CSF sediment is negative; (2) CSF CIE for bacterial pathogens, if available, is negative; (3) the patient does not appear extremely toxic nor have signs of grossly altered consciousness; (4) CSF white blood count is <2000/mm³ and protein is <200 mg percent and glucose is >35 mg percent. It has been shown that during this 6–8 hour observation period the CSF pleocytosis will usually shift from polymorphonuclear to predominantly mononuclear cells. Such a shift strongly supports the clinical impression of a non-bacterial infection. While awaiting the 6–8 hours to repeat the lumbar puncture, if the patient deteriorates clinically, therapy should be started promptly with ampicillin, or alternately with penicillin or chloramphenicol.

Patients with Known Predisposition to Meningitis

If microbial meningitis of unknown etiology develops in a patient with a particular predisposition to infection, the initial antimicrobial regimen must be chosen with knowledge of the organisms that commonly cause infection in that predisposing situation (Table 12-3). These predispositions include: (1) head trauma, (2) neurosurgical procedures, (3) anatomic defects in the cranium or spine, (4) head and neck carcinomas, (5) contiguous infections, (6) immunosuppression, and (7) miscellaneous underlying conditions such as endocarditis, alcoholism, and drug addiction.

In patients with meningitis occurring within three days of non-penetrating, non-depressed head trauma, *S. pneumoniae* is the most common pathogen. Penicillin alone is adequate therapy. With open or penetrating head injury or with meningitis developing five days after non-penetrating trauma, infection caused by skin flora (*S. aureus* and aerobic gram-negative bacilli) should be suspected and initial therapy must be broad-spectrum including a penicillinase-resistant penicillin (i.e., nafcillin), chloramphenicol, and an aminoglycoside. Intrathecal aminoglycoside therapy frequently cannot be administered in this setting, but should be considered if the patient is seriously ill or deteriorates clinically despite intravenous therapy. Patients with a CSF rhinorrhea or basilar skull fracture or dural tears are especially prone to pneumococcal meningitis.[41]

Meningitis developing after a neurosurgical procedure or in association with some other breach in cranial (or spinal) anatomic barriers (head and neck carcinomas, congenital defects) needs an initial antibiotic regimen effective against skin flora (staphylococci, gram-negative bacilli, streptococci). Intravenous nafcillin, gentamicin, and chloramphenicol would be appropriate. When otitis, sinusitis, or mastoiditis is associated with meningitis, initial therapy should cover *S. pneumoniae* and *H. influenzae* as well as *S. aureus* and gram-negative bacilli since the focus may be chronic rather than acute. Nafcillin, chloramphenicol and gentamicin are appropriate.

Patients with altered immune response due to malignant neoplasm or immunosuppressive drug therapy are at risk for developing a wide range of bacterial, fungal, and parasitic meningitides.[10] Bacterial infection is most common. When the causative agent has not been identified, initial therapy must include drugs active against the common bacterial pathogens (*S. pneumoniae*, *N. meningitidis*) but also against *L. monocytogenes* and gram-negative bacilli. The latter organisms are frequent in granulocytopenic patients, while Listeria occurs most frequently in patients with depressed cellular immunity such as those with lymphoma or renal transplant. Cryptococcal infections are also common in these two groups of immunosuppressed patients, while staphylococcal meningitis is not. In immunosuppressed patients, an initial regimen of penicillin (or ampicillin) and chloramphenicol and gentamicin is appropriate. Carbenicillin should probably be added in granulocytopenic patients. If the patient does not respond clinically, an empiric trial of intravenous amphotericin B should be considered.

Partially Treated Bacterial Meningitis

Patients with meningitis who have received antibiotic therapy prior to admission, present diagnostic and therapeutic problems.[16,27,29] The chance that one or two days of oral antibiotics will convert CSF findings typical of bacterial meningitis to those resembling an aseptic process has been exaggerated. Recent evidence indicates that partial treatment reduces the percentage of positive CSF Gram's stains and cultures by about 30 percent. In less than 10 percent of cases are the CSF findings so altered as to provide no evidence suggesting a bacterial process, and most of these patients had received prolonged therapy.

When faced with the problem of a patient with acute meningitis who has already received antibiotic treatment and whose CSF Gram's stain is negative, the potential usefulness of rapid serologic diagnostic techniques should not be overlooked. These include CIE (*S. pneumoniae*, *N. meningiditis*, *H. influenzae*), the limulus endotoxin assay (gram-negative bacilli), and CSF lactate levels (increased in bacterial infections). If positive, any of these three tests strongly suggest presence of a bacterial infection and indicate the need for antibiotic therapy. Like other laboratory procedures, these tests are not foolproof, however. There is some convincing data which suggests that antibiotic therapy can safely be withheld in an alert patient with the following CSF values on initial LP: WBC < 1200/mm^3; glucose > 40 mg percent; protein < 150 mg percent.[27] In many situations patients with partially treated meningitis must be committed to a 10–14 day course of antibiotics because their physicians are understandably unable to decide whether the negative CSF smears and cultures resulted from prior treatment or a nonbacterial infection. Such empiric courses of chloramphenicol or ampicillin are the prudent approach in uncertain situations.

BRAIN ABSCESS

General Considerations

The management of brain abscess differs substantially from management of meningitis because of the essential role which neurosurgery plays in diagnosis and therapy. Since the introduction of modern antibiotic therapy, brain abscess must be treated more as an expanding mass lesion than as a potentially fatal source of central nervous system sepsis. The advent of potent antimicrobial agents and the increasing sophistication of neurosurgery have not substantially decreased the morbidity and mortality associated with brain abscesses.[7, 36] Optimal prognosis for patients with brain abscesses can only be provided by early suspicion of the diagnosis, rapid diagnostic evaluation, and prompt medical and surgical treatment.[24]

Brain abscesses are caused by spread of infection from contiguous foci of suppuration, hematogenous spread from distant foci of infection, or mechanical breach of the subarachnoid space. The location of the abscess frequently suggests the source of infection.[4,7,8,11] Frontal lobe abscesses commonly arise from chronic frontal sinus infection. Temporal lobe and cerebellar abscesses arise from chronic middle ear or mastoid infections. Multiple cerebral abscesses are frequently due to hematogenous spread from pleural, pulmonary, or pelvic sources, especially in patients with congenital heart disease and right to left shunts. Dental abscesses and endocarditis are less frequent causes.[22]

Infection spreads to the brain from contiguous foci either by direct extension or retrograde passage along venous channels.[4] Hematogenous spread is caused by deposition of infected emboli in small vessels. The inflammation caused by organisms within brain parenchyma destroys brain tissue and causes adjacent edema. Edema can have drastic consequences by causing the cerebral or cerebellar structures to herniate compressing vital areas of the midbrain. The initial alteration caused by infection in the brain substance is hemorrhagic infarction. The involved tissue is hyperemic with necrotic blood vessels and extravasated erythrocytes. The maturation of the local response is important for optimal surgical evacuation of the abscess. Fibroblasts migrate from blood vessel walls, and a fibrous capsule forms around the inflammatory mass. This fibrous capsule forms more rapidly on the lateral or gray surface of the cortex, probably due to that area's extensive vascularity. Thus abscesses tend to penetrate centripetally rather than centrifugally. The inflammatory reaction may or may not involve adjacent leptomeninges.

Brain abscesses may present in subtle ways. While many patients have headache and fever and focal neurologic signs, brain abscesses should be suspected even if these cardinal manifestations are absent. A patient with apparent meningitis should be suspected of having a brain abscess if he develops focal neurologic signs, focal seizures, or papilledema. The presence of congenital heart disease with shunt, bronchiectasis, lung abscess, pleural empyema, or a history of neurosurgery or trauma in a patient with meningitis should also raise the suspicion of abscess. The isolation from the CSF of multiple organisms, or of individual organisms other than *N. meningitidis, H. influenzae,* or *S. pneumoniae* should also arouse suspicion of an abscess.[12] CNS infection with focal neurologic signs in an immunosuppressed patient, particularly patients with acute leukemia, should suggest abscess.

Diagnosis of a brain abscess can be established by radioisotope scan, computer assisted tomography (CAT), or arteriography.[4,7,8,21,36] The brain scan and CAT scan are quite sensitive, documenting lesions of 1 cm or less, and are particularly valuable for documenting multiple lesions. The radioisotope scan cannot distinguish cerebritis from abscess. Neither scanning technique can reliably distinguish abscess from hemorrhage or tumor. Arteriography can define the mass lesion, provides information useful for distinguishing the lesion from tumor or hemorrhage, and may be able to define the abscess capsule. The abscess capsule can also be visualized by CAT scan. The definition of the capsule can be an important determinant of the optimal time for neurosurgical treatment in a stable and alert patient.

Lumbar puncture should not be done if a brain abscess is documented or suspected.[36] Bacteriology of CSF is usually negative or incomplete, and herniation is a common complication. It is preferable to start empiric antimicrobial therapy while evaluating the patient rather than risk devastating and irreversible brain-stem damage by performing a lumbar puncture.

Management of Brain Abscess

Since increased intracranial pressure and resulting compression of vital brain-stem centers are the primary causes of morbidity and mortality in brain abscesses, decompression of the lesion is the most important part of effective therapy. Pharmacologic agents which decrease cerebral edema, prevent seizures, and eradicate the microorganisms are important aspects of management, but surgical evacuation of the abscess is of utmost importance.

While management must be directed toward prompt recognition and surgical treatment to prevent herniation, premature neurosurgery should be avoided since early, poorly encapsulated lesions are difficult or impossible to drain or excise, and a second neurosurgical procedure may become necessary.

A patient with signs of herniation and midbrain compression, deteriorating mental status, or evidence of abscess rupture into the ventricles must have the abscess evacuated. Antimicrobial agents, osmotic diuretics, and steroids must be administered concomitantly while the necessary diagnostic tests and surgical preparations are carried out. Abscess drainage is the only effective means of preserving neurologic function in this urgent situation.[4,17]

A fully alert patient with a stable neurologic deficit and no signs of increased intracranial pressure can undergo full diagnostic work-up while receiving empiric antimicrobial therapy. After 7–10 days a capsule will usually form around the abscess and can be demonstrated by CAT scan or arteriogram. An elective evacuation of the abscess can then be performed.

Medical Decompression

Medical decompression of the brain for patients with increased intracranial pressure has a useful role in the acutely ill patient but cannot replace surgical intervention. Patients with brain abscesses can present with signs of midbrain compression or apparently stable patients can precipitously deteriorate. In these emergent situations, decompression with osmotic agents is probably beneficial. Mannitol (25–30 g) should be given by an intravenous bolus. This dose may be repeated every 4–6 hours or a continuous infusion maintained (25–50 g every 4 hours) while the patient is undergoing emergency diagnostic procedures and preparation for surgery. Glycerol can also be used, but has not been extensively evaluated. It has the disadvantage in the preoperative patient of requiring oral administration.

Glucocorticosteroids decrease cerebral edema by inhibiting inflammatory response, and are important in the medical therapy of increased intracranial pressure.[32] Their onset of action is slow (4–8 hours). The relative disadvantages of their anti-inflammatory action in terms of inhibition of capsule formation around the abscess are uncertain. Prednisone (5–25 mg intravenously every 6 hours) or dexamethasone (4 mg intravenously every 6 hours), can be given.

Antimicrobial Therapy

General Considerations. Effective antimicrobial therapy is essential to complete resolution of a brain abscess. The antibiotic chosen must penetrate the abscess well and should be chosen with knowledge of the sensitivity pattern of the known or suspected organisms. Careful microbiologic studies of the abscess contents, including aerobic and anaerobic cultures for bacteria, cultures for fungi and mycobacteria and stains for bacteria, fungi, mycobacteria, and (when indicated) protozoa should always be done. The antibiotic sensitivity patterns of the specific organisms should be determined by a quantitative method.

Drug penetration into CSF is not identical to penetration into brain substance. Chloramphenicol is the only drug which reaches high levels in brain parenchyma: the parenchyma to blood concentration ratios can be as high as 9:11.[26] Penicillin, ampicillin, and cephalothin all have low ratios (1:7 or less) when normal brain tissue is analyzed. Local inflammation may enhance the concentration of an antibiotic in brain tissue. With inflammation, penicillin and ampicillin have been found to reach effective concentrations in an abscess. Penetration of all antibiotics is erratic, however. Thus to maximize the likelihood of attaining effective local antibiotic concentrations, high doses of antibiotic should be given parenterally. Table 11-7 indicates the recommended drugs and dosages when the specific organisms are known. If the abscess contains more than one organism, multiple antibiotics may be necessary. Table 11-5 indicates recommended drugs and dosage when a presumptive diagnosis of brain abscess has been made but specific organisms have not been isolated.

The duration of antimicrobial therapy necessary to sterilize brain tissue adjacent to an excised or drained abscess has not been established.[11,22,26] The duration of treatment must be determined for each patient individually. Systemic antimicrobial therapy should be given for at least 4 weeks. A slow clinical response to therapy or failure of the lesion to resolve rapidly as judged by isotope scan, CAT, or radiographs of the contrast filled cavity should encourage longer courses of therapy.

Basic principles of the choice of antimicrobial therapy have been discussed earlier in this chapter.

Local instillation of antibiotics into abscess cavities has not been shown to be effective, and should never be used without systemic therapy. Local antibiotic instillation can cause inflammation and seizures. Intrathecal administration of antibiotics has no role in the therapy of abscess since the antibiotic is unlikely to penetrate into the abscess from the CSF.

Initial antimicrobial therapy   of brain abscess must encompass a considerably broader spectrum than initial therapy of meningitis. While most cases of meningitis are caused by only one of a fairly predictable group of organisms, brain abscesses are caused usually by multiple and diverse microorganisms.[12] In meningitis, gram stain or CIE of the CSF frequently identifies the organism with near certainty very soon after the patient comes to medical attention. Such information is rarely available with brain abscesses, and initial therapy must be guided by knowledge of the apparent pathogenesis of the infection, and the spectrum of organisms typically encountered with that etiologic process. Frontal lobe abscesses found with nasal sinus infection are commonly due to aerobic and anaerobic streptococci, pneumococci, and occasionally *H. influenzae.* Ampicillin or chloramphenicol alone is adequate initial therapy.

Temporal lobe or cerebellar abscesses due to middle ear or mastoid infection commonly are caused by aerobic and anaerobic streptococci, but also by *S. aureus* and gram-negative bacilli.[12,40] In this situation nafcillin and gentamicin should be added to chloramphenicol for the initial regimen. Addition of carbenicillin or ticarcillin therapy should also be considered if a Gram's stain of ear discharge shows many gram-negative bacilli or Pseudomonas is known to be present in the ear discharge.

Brain abscesses occurring in patients who have had recent neurosurgery or trauma are frequently caused by skin flora such as *S. aureus* and *B. hemolytic streptococci,* and gram-negative bacilli, with the latter particularly seen in hospitalized patients.

Brain abscesses in patients with known extracranial infection or bacteremia should be treated with consideration of the known extracranial organisms. It should be kept in mind that the organism isolated from blood may not represent all the organisms which seeded the brain from a lung abscess or some other source.

Brain abscesses of unknown origin should be treated with intravenous chloramphenicol alone. If the patient is immunosuppressed, particularly a leukopenic patient with acute leukemia, gentamicin and carbenicillin should be added initially since gram-negative bacilli are frequent pathogens. If the patient is moribund or does not respond to treatment while awaiting neurosurgery, consideration must be given to the addition of systemic amphotericin B since cryptococcal abscesses are not uncommon in immunosuppressed patients.

Definitive Antibiotic Regimen.   The efficacy of individual drugs for the treatment of brain abscess is not as well established as their efficacy for meningitis. The influence of cerebral edema, herniation, and neurosurgery on outcome make evaluation of specific antibiotics difficult. Table 11-7 lists the drugs of choice when specific organisms are suspected or identified.

Debridement of Contiguous Foci.   A large number of brain abscesses are associated with contiguous infection. In addition to neurosurgical decompression and antimicrobial therapy, eradication of the contiguous focus is essential. Patients must be carefully assessed for sinus or middle ear infection prior to neurosurgery. If a contiguous suppurative infection is present, it should be treated surgically as soon as technically feasible.

Anticonvulsant Therapy.　Patients with supratentorial brain abscesses have a high incidence of focal and generalized seizures. Diazepam 5–10 mg intravenously can be used to terminate continuous or repetitive seizures. Prolonged anticonvulsant therapy should be given to all patients after surgical procedure to treat supratentorial abscess and to any patient who had seizures prior to neurosurgery. Phenytoin is the preferred anticonvulsant. See chapter on management of seizure disorders.

Long Term Management.　During the post-operative period, and after cessation of antimicrobial therapy, the patient's neurologic status should be carefully followed. Progression of focal neurologic defects or deterioration of the patient's level of consciousness should prompt reevaluation of the patient. Recurrence of the abscess should be considered, particularly if the lesion was drained rather than excised, as well as the possibility of a second or third abscess that originally escaped detection. The infected area should be evaluated post-operatively by CAT scan if possible. Isotope scans and plain skull roentgenograms (if contrast material was placed in the cavity at the time of surgery) are less desirable methods for assessing resolution. Glucocorticosteroids should be tapered rapidly in the immediate post-operative period. Phenytoin should be continued for 1–2 years with supratentorial abscesses, or longer if the EEG is focally abnormal.

There is no role for oral antibiotics following completion of the 4–6 week course of parenteral therapy.

Complications of brain abscess must be watched for, including noncommunicating hydrocephalus (particularly if rupture into the ventricles occurred) and inappropriate ADH secretion (Table 11-4). If the patient has residual neurologic deficits, reversible causes such as hydrocephalus, drug toxicity, or subdural hematoma must be considered.

SUBDURAL EMPYEMA

Subdural empyema is a localized pyogenic infection which develops in the subdural space. The causative infection commonly spreads from the frontal sinuses, and less frequently from chronic otitis media, penetrating head trauma, or subarachnoid infection.[25,45,47] Hematogenous spread of microorganisms to sterile subdural hematomas also occurs. Subdural empyema is similar to a brain abscess in its pathogenesis, bacteriology, and treatment. Morbidity and mortality is related to increased intracranial pressure and resulting herniation, cortical venous phlebitis, and spread to dural sinuses or brain parenchyma. Subdural empyema should be suspected in a patient with clinical evidence of a CNS infection and either papilledema, focal seizures, or hemiparesis even if the brain scan is normal. Since empyema can spread under the falx, bilateral involvement is not uncommon. The bacterial flora found are similar to that for brain abscesses and usually consist of both aerobic and anaerobic organisms.

Patient management is similar to that for brain abscess. Surgical decompression is an urgent consideration when signs of increased intracranial pressure are present. Bilateral involvement must be sought either at surgery or by pre-operative arteriography.

Because of the rarity of subdural empyemas, little information is available about the penetration of antibiotics into subdural empyemas. Drugs which penetrate inflamed meninges seem most likely to be beneficial. Empiric antibiotic therapy is influenced by the likely source of infection. Intravenous antimicrobial therapy should be continued for a minimum of 3–4 weeks. Longer therapy may be dictated by slow clinical response. Reaccumulation of pus or sterile fluid must be watched for by careful neurologic examination and CAT scanning. The only indication for local installation of antibiotic is resistance of the organism to all drugs which penetrate inflamed meninges. Even in this situation, the efficacy and safety of local irrigation is unknown. Anticonvulsants are given prophylactically to prevent seizures.

SPINAL EPIDURAL ABSCESS

Spinal epidural abscesses are uncommon, but prompt diagnosis and therapy are needed to avoid irreversible damage due to spinal cord compression. Trauma, operative contamination, contiguous bone or soft tissue infection, and hematogenous spread are the common sources of this infection.[1] *S. aureus* is the most often isolated organism.[37] Gram-negative bacilli, however, cause a substantial fraction of infections. Studies to date have shown anaerobes to be uncommon.

Like brain abscess and subdural abscess, surgical decompression is essential if irreversible spinal cord damage is to be avoided. Laminectomy with exposure of the entire longitudinal extent of the abscess should be performed in order to assure adequate drainage. Antimicrobial therapy is directed toward the organisms cultured at the time of surgery. Presumptive treatment should include nafcillin or oxacillin with an aminoglycoside. Antimicrobial treatment should be continued intravenously for at least 4 weeks, and for 6–8 weeks if osteomyelitis is present. The patient's neurologic status must be followed carefully after stopping antibiotics. Spine films should be obtained periodically after initiation of therapy to rule out osteomyelitis. Bone scanning may be useful in assessing the presence of osteomyelitis before radiologically detected lesions can be recognized. Considerable skill is needed to differentiate postoperative changes from infection.

ENCEPHALITIS

Although the syndromes of encephalitis or meningoencephalitis are usually equated with viral infections, it is important to note that almost any infectious agent may on occasion produce these syndromes. Examples include parasitic and spirochetal infections, bacterial endocarditis, rickettsial diseases, and *Mycoplasma pneumoniae*. Therapy for these infections has already been presented.

With the exception of encephalitis caused by *Herpes simplex (H. hominis)* and perhaps that associated with disseminated varicella-zoster virus infection in immunosuppressed patients, there is no specific or effective therapy available for the viral agents capable of causing encephalitis. Trials with antiviral drugs such as idoxuridine (IUDR), and cytosine arabinoside (ARA-C) have demonstrated that they are toxic and ineffective. Importantly, however, it has recently been shown in a controlled study that vidarabine (ARA-A) is both efficacious and nontoxic in the treatment of *H. simplex* encephalitis.[46] To have a beneficial effect, vidarabine must be given early in the course of infection, before the onset of coma. Sporadic data suggest that ARA-A may also be effective for encephalitis caused by disseminated *Herpes zoster*.

MISCELLANEOUS SYSTEMIC INFECTIONS INVOLVING THE CNS

Poliomyelitis

Poliomyelitis is an acute viral illness caused by three antigenically related viruses which involve both the meninges as well as the motor neurons of the brain-stem and spinal cord. Polio virus infection may be inapparent, but can cause aseptic meningitis or irreversible paralysis. There is no therapy, except supportive treatment for muscle spasm, paralysis, and respiratory failure.

Rabies

Rabies is a progressive paralytic disease, usually ending in death. The virus is introduced by implantation by a bite or scratch. Specific chemotherapy is not available once overt rabies occurs. Vigilant supportive care has resulted in survival in rare instances.

Tetanus

Tetanus is a disorder of neuromuscular function which is caused by a potent toxin elaborated by *Clostridium tetani.* These organisms are found in contaminated wounds or other deep tissue infections. The toxin reaches the CNS and suppresses inhibitory influences on motor neurons and interneurons. Therapy is based on attentive supportive care, neutralization of toxin, and removal of the source of toxin. Muscle relaxants such as diazepam or meprobamate are almost always needed for sedation and relief of muscle rigidity. Patients often must be treated for days or weeks with a neuromuscular blocking agent such as curare or pavulon, and provided with mechanical respiratory assistance. For patients with clinical tetanus, human derived tetanus immune globulin should be administered immediately in a dose of 3000 units injected intramuscularly at three different sites. Further administration of immune globulin is unnecessary. If human immune globulin is unavailable, 10,000 units of horse antitoxin can be given after a small subcutaneous test dose to exclude hypersensitivity. Active immunization should be started immediately with intramuscular alum-adsorbed toxoid followed by a second dose 1–2 months later and a third dose 6–12 months later. Any wound which could be a likely source of the Clostridium, should be thoroughly debrided and left open. Adequate debridement makes antimicrobial therapy unnecessary, but high doses of penicillin G (24,000,000 units per day) are usually given intravenously. A cephalosporin or tetracycline is used for penicillin allergic patients.

Rickettsial Diseases

Rickettsial diseases include epidemic typhus (*Rickettsia prowazekii*), endemic or Murine typhus (*R. mooseri*), rickettsialpox (*R. akari*), tsutsugamushi disease or scrub typhus (*R. tsutsugamushi*), rocky mountain spotted fever (*R. rickettsii*), and several tick borne fevers of the Eastern hemisphere (*R. conorri, R. australis, R. siberica*). Central nervous system manifestations can be prominent in each of the rickettsial diseases. The clinical picture most often resembles encephalitis but signs of meningeal irritation are common. Antimicrobials are effective in treating all of the above varieties of Rickettsial disease and the agent of choice is chloramphenicol or tetracycline.

Tularemia

Francisella tularensis is transmitted to man by arthropod vectors or infected animal tissue. Meningitis or encephalitis may be manifestations of tularemia. Streptomycin is the drug of choice for systemic tularemia, but because of its poor penetration into the CNS, infection of brain parenchyma or the meninges require treatment with chloramphenicol or tetracycline.

REFERENCES

1. Baker AS, Ojemann RG, Swartz MN, Richardson EP: Spinal epidural abscess. N Engl J Med 293: 463–468, 1975.
2. Barret-Connor E: Tuberculous meningitis in adults. South Med J 60: 1061–1067, 1967.
3. Bayer AS, Seidel JS, Yoshikawa TT, Anthony BF, Grore LB: Groys D. Enterococcal meningitis. Arch Intern Med 136: 883–886, 1976.
4. Beller AJ, Sahar A, Praiss I: Brain abscess—Review of 89 cases over a period of 30 years. J Neurol Neurosurg Psych 36: 757–768, 1973.
5. Bennett JE: Chemotherapy of systemic mycoses. N Engl J Med 289: 30–32, 320–322, 1974.
6. Bobrowitz ID: Ethambutol in tuberculous meningitis. Chest 61: 629–632, 1972.
7. Brewer NS, MacCarty CS, Wellman WE: Brain abscess: a review of recent experience. Ann Intern Med 82: 571–576, 1975.
8. Carey ME, Chou SN, French LA: Experience with brain abscesses. J Neurosurg 36: 1–9, 1972.
9. Carpenter RR, Petersdorf RG: The clinical spectrum of bacterial meningitis. Amer J Med 33: 262–275, 1962.
10. Chernik NL, Armstrong D, Posner JB: Central nervous system infections in patients with cancer. Medicine 52: 563–581, 1973.
11. Delouvois J, Gortvai P, Hurley R: Antibiotic treatment of abscesses of the central nervous system. BMJ 2: 985–987, 1977.
12. DeLouvois J, Gortvai P, Hurley R: Bacteriology of abscesses of the central nervous system: a multicentre prospective study. BMJ 2: 981–984, 1977.
13. Deresinski SC, Lilly RB, Levine HB, Gralgiani JN, Stevens DA: Treatment of fungal meningitis with miconazole. Arch Intern Med 137: 1180–1185, 1977.
14. Diamond RD, Bennett JE: A subcutaneous reservoir for intrathecal therapy of fungal meningitis. N Engl J Med 288: 186–188, 1973.
15. D'Oliverira JJG: Cerebrospinal fluid concentrations of rifampin in meningeal tuberculosis. Amer Rev Resp Dis 106: 432–437, 1972.
16. Editorial: Partly treated pyogenic meningitis. Brit Med J 1: 340, 1977.
17. Garfield J: Management of supratentorial intracranial abscess: A review of 200 cases. BMJ 2: 7–11, 1969.
18. Gilles FH, Jammes JL, Berenberg W: Neonatal meningitis. The ventricle as a bacterial reservoir. Arch Neurol 34: 560–562, 1977.
19. Hambleton G, Davies PA: Diagnosis and management of bacterial meningitis. Drug 8: 15–53, 1974.
20. Hawley HB, Gump DW: Vancomycin therapy of bacterial meningitis. Amer J Dis Child 126: 261–264, 1973.
21. Heineman HS, Braude AI, Osterholm JL: Intracranial suppurative disease—early presumptive diagnosis and successful treatment without surgery. JAMA 218: 1542–1547, 1971.
22. Ingham HR, Selkon JB, Roxby CM: Bacteriologic study of otogenic cerebral abscesses: chemotherapeutic role of metronidazole. BMJ 2: 991–993, 1977.

23. KAISER AB, McGEE ZA: Aminoglycoside therapy of gram-negative bacillary meningitis. N Engl J Med 293: 1215–1220, 1975.
24. KARANDANIS D, SHULMAN JA: Factors associated with mortality in brain abscess. Arch Intern Med 135: 1145–1150, 1975.
25. KAUFMAN DM, MILLER MH, STEIGBIGEL NH: Subdural empyema: Analysis of 17 recent cases and review of the literature. Medicine 54: 485–498, 1975.
26. KRAMER PW, GRIFFITH RS, CAMPBELL RL: Antibiotic penetration of the brain—a comparative study. J Neurosurg 31: 295–302, 1969.
27. LEON-VALIENTE C, RAMIREZ-RONDA CH: Partially treated meningitis in adults, a prospective study (abstract). 16th Interscience Conference on Antimicrobial Agents and Chemotherapy, Chicago, p 242, 1976.
28. LERNER PI: Selection of antimicrobial agents in bacterial infections of the nervous system. Adv Neurol 6: 169–203, 1974.
29. MANDAL BK: The dilemma of partially treated bacterial meningitis. Scand J Infect Dis 8: 185–188, 1976.
30. MOHR JA, GRIFFITHS W, JACKSON R, SAADAH H, BIRD P, RIDDLE J: Neurosyphilis and penicillin levels in cerebrospinal fluid. JAMA 236: 2208–2209, 1976.
31. NEWBERRY WM: Drug treatment of the systemic mycoses. Semin Drug Treat 2: 313–329, 1972.
32. QUARTEY CRC, JOHNSTON JA, ROZDILSKY B: Decadron in the treatment of cerebral abscess. J Neurosurg 45: 301–310, 1976.
33. RAHAL JJ: Treatment of gram-negative bacillary meningitis in adults. Ann Intern Med 77: 295–302, 1972.
34. RAHAL JJ, HYAMS PJ, SIMBERCOFF MS, RUBINSTEIN E: Combined intrathecal and intramuscular gentamycin for gram-negative meningitis. N Engl J Med 290: 1394–1398, 1974.
35. ROOT TE, HARRIS AA, LEVIN S: Diagnosis and treatment of tuberculous and fungal meningitis. In: Clinical Neuropharmacology, (ed: Klawans HL) Raven Press, New York, 1977.
36. SAMSON DS, CLARK K: A current review of brain abscess. Am J Med 54: 201–210, 1973.
37. SCHLOSSBERG D, SHULMAN JA: Spinal epidural abscess. S Med J 70: 669–673, 1977.
38. SCHORNBAUM SC, GARDNER P, SHILLITO J: Infections of cerebrospinal fluid shunts: epidemiology, clinical manifestations, and therapy. J Infect Dis 131: 543–552, 1975.
39. SHACKELFORD PG, BOBINSKI JE, FEIGIN RD, CHERRY JD: Therapy of Haemophilus influenzae meningitis reconsidered. N Engl J Med 287: 634–638, 1972.
40. SHAW MDM, RUSSELL JA: Cerebellar abscess—a review of 47 cases. J Neurol Neurosurg Psychiat 38: 429–435, 1975.
41. SWARTZ MN, DODGE PR: Bacterial meningitis—a review of selected aspects. N Engl J Med 272: 725–731, 779–787, 842–848, 898–902, 954–960, 1003–1010, 1965.
42. TRAMONT EC: Persistence of treponema pallidum following penicillin G therapy. JAMA 236: 2206–2207, 1976.
43. UTZ JP: Current and future chemotherapy of central nervous system fungal infections. Adv Neurol 6: 127–132, 1974.

44. Utz JP, Grarriques IL, Sande MA, Warner JF, Mandell CL, McGehee RF, Duma RJ, Shadomy S: Therapy of cryptococcosis with a combination of flucytosine and amphotercin B. J Infect Dis 132: 368–373, 1975.
45. Van Alphen HAM, Dreissen JJR: Brain abscess and subdural empyema—factors influencing mortality and results of various surgical techniques. J Neurol Neurosurg Psych 39: 481–490, 1976.
46. Whitley RJ, Soong SJ, Dolin R, Calasso GJ, Ch'ien LT, Alford CA: Adenine arabinoside therapy of biopsy-proven Herpes simplex encephalitis. N Engl J Med 297: 289–294, 1977.
47. Yoshikawa TT, Chow AW, Cuze LB: Role of anaerobic bacteria in subdural empyema—report of four cases and review of 327 cases from the English literature. Am J Med 58: 99–104, 1975.

12

Drug-Induced Disorders of the Nervous System

USE OF DRUGS IN THE PRESENCE OF ASSOCIATED NEUROLOGICAL DISEASES

If certain drugs are used in the presence of nervous system disorders, aggravation of existing symptoms may occur or new symptoms may be induced. Therefoe, one must always consider the potential neurotoxicity of drugs prescribed for the patient with neurological diseases.[3]

Myasthenia Gravis and Other Neuromuscular Disorders

In patients with myasthenia gravis, certain drugs may increase the muscle weakness, especially in those with generalized severe myasthenia.[4,7] Most likely to exert such effect are the polymyxin antibiotics such as colistin and polymyxin B and the aminoglycoside antibiotics gentamicin, kanamycin and streptomycin. A dilemma often exists in patients with myasthenia gravis: severe infection is a threat to the patient but antibiotics pose a hazard as well. If it is decided to use antibiotics that may adversely affect the myasthenia symptoms, one must be prepared to deal with the increase in weakness, including respiratory paralysis; and avoid excessive doses of antibiotics.

Migraine and Other Disorders

Progesteron-estrogen contraceptive agents may sometimes aggravate the attacks in patients with migraine headaches. Therefore they should be used with caution.

Drugs with depressant action on respiration such as barbiturates and opiate analgesics can be hazardous, particularly in the presence of increased intracranial pressure due to cerebral tumors or trauma. They may raise the intracranial pressure further by inducing cerebral vasodilatation as a consequence of carbon dioxide retention from the respiratory depression.[3]

Toxic delirium is often induced by drugs in patients with degenerative neurological disorders, which is discussed further under the section on Nervous system disorders induced by drugs.

Aggravation of seizures in epileptic patients by drugs that can cause seizures per se may occur, but is generally rare.

NERVOUS SYSTEM DISORDERS INDUCED BY DRUGS

Disorders of nervous system induced by drugs may involve both the central and peripheral nervous system. Among the clinical manifestations are diffuse encephalopathies, cerebrovascular syndromes, extrapyramidal and cerebellar syndromes, myelopathies, peripheral neuropathies and neuromuscular syndromes. The neurological disorders induced by drugs are particularly prone to occur in elderly individuals and in those with impaired renal function.

Toxic Delirium

One of the most frequently occurring neurological disorders induced by drugs is toxic delirium.[1,2] This is characterized by confusion, disorientation, anxiety, delusions and sometimes hallucinations. It is common in older patients, patients with dementia and cerebral atrophy or in patients with degenerative CNS diseases. The causative agents include sedatives, reserpine, methyldopa, alcohol, digitalis, anticholinergics, tricyclic antidepressants, antianxiety and antipsychotic drugs. Stopping the causative medication usually reverses the process, but it may take several weeks before mental processes fully recover.

Convulsions

Convulsions may be induced by central nervous system stimulants and analeptics such as amphetamines and bemegride. Penicillin G (often used in the laboratory to produce experimental seizures in animals) may cause convulsions in patients with relatively small amounts, such as 50,000 units, when applied intrathecally or intracerebrally for infections.[1,2] Penicillin encephalopathy, characterized by confusion, stupor and multifocal myoclonus, culminating in generalized convulsions may be caused by intravenously administered, massive daily doses of penicillin (over 25 million units). This is likely to occur particularly in elderly patients with impaired renal function or in those undergoing cardiac surgery with cardio-pulmonary bypass. Myoclonic seizures have also been noted in patients treated with high doses of cephalosporins intravenously. Other antimicrobial agents that may cause convulsions are cycloserine and isoniazid.[6] Convulsions caused by isoniazid are probably due to pyridoxine deficiency and are most likely to occur in those who are genetically slow inactivators of isoniazid. The urinary antiseptic nalidixic acid has been reported to exacerbate seizures in epileptic patients or after excessive doses in non-epileptics; renal impairment may make this complication more likely to occur.

Local anesthetic agents such as procaine and lidocaine when applied locally in high concentrations or accidentally injected intravenously have caused seizures, as have excessive doses of lidocaine when used in the treatment of cardiac arrhythmias. Other agents that have been noted on rare occasions to cause convulsions or aggravate the seizures in epileptic patients include insulin, phenothiazines, MAO inhibitors, antihistamines, tricyclic antidepressants, chloroquine, vincristine and oral contraceptives.[2]

Extrapyramidal Syndromes

Extrapyramidal signs and symptoms may be caused by agents that block or deplete the brain catecholamines or serotonin.[2] Among those are phenothiazines, Rauwolfia alkaloids and other psychotropic drugs such as butyrophenones (haloperidol) and thioxanthenes (thiothixene). A frequently occurring clinical picture is akathisia characterized by motor restlessness causing the patient to pace about or tap his feet and shift the legs often while sitting. Often present are grimacing, smacking of lips and tongue and chewing movements. A parkinsonian-like state may also occur, usually starting with tremor, followed by rigidity and motor retardation. Dyskinesias mostly of dystonic type with twisting, writhing movements, torticollis and oculogyric crises are not infrequent.

These drug-induced extrapyramidal manifestations tend to be more severe in patients who receive higher doses and they tend to occur more frequently in females than in males, but some patients seem to be inherently more susceptible than others. Age seems to play a role in that older patients tend to develop a parkinsonian-like state and younger patients a dystonic picture, which can be confused with encephalitis or tetanus in children who have taken overdoses of phenothiazines. Acute dystonic reactions can also be caused by antiemetic metoclopramide, particularly in children after administration of large doses.

The drug-induced extrapyramidal signs and symptoms, with rare exceptions, are reversible after discontinuation or reduction of the dosage of the causative agent, but permanent or tardive dyskinesias have been reported. If the drug must be continued in a dosage that is causing symptoms, amelioration can often be achieved with antihistamines and antiparkinsonian drugs and possibly with pimozide or tetrabenazine.

Drug-Induced Complications Related to Cerebral Circulation

Among the complications related to the cerebral circulation are intracerebral or subarachnoidal hemorrhages following hypertensive crises caused by monoamine oxidase inhibitors, when these drugs are given together with tyramine-rich foods or sympathomimetic drugs. Intracerebral hemorrhages may also occur as a result of poorly controlled anticoagulant therapy or with the administration of pressor amines such as adrenaline and noradrenaline, particularly in patients with intracerebral aneurysms or clotting defects. Cerebral infarctions have been reported resulting from a sudden fall of blood pressure induced by ganglion blocking antihypertensive drugs such as pentolinium and hexamethonium.

Oral contraceptives have been associated with reports of intracranial arterial thrombosis or embolus, as well as sinus thrombosis.[2]

Encephalopathy and Other Brain Syndromes

Vaccines and antisera may cause encephalomyelitis, particularly the smallpox and pertussis vaccine and tetanus antitoxin.[1,2] Excessive dosage of lithium carbonate may lead to neurological manifestations such as coma, spasticity, convulsions, particularly in the presence of impaired renal function.

Slurred speech, confusion and coma have occurred with the use of usual doses of lidocaine in patients with severe liver impairment. In patients with liver failure, encephalopathy may be precipitated or aggravated by opiates or overvigorous therapy with diuretic agents. Encephalopathy can also be caused by methotrexate and 1-asparaginase.

A number of drugs can lead to the syndrome of pseudotumor cerebri which is characterized by headache, blurred vision, increased intracranial pressure and papilledema. In this respect corticosteroids, especially in children or when used in high doses in adults, as well as excessive dosage of vitamin A are most commonly implicated. Oral contraceptives and the use of nalidixic acid and tetracyclines in infants have also been incriminated on a few occasions. A cerebral syndrome manifested by headaches, drowsiness and vertigo may be caused by indomethacin.

Cerebellar Syndromes

High doses of antiepileptic drugs often cause cerebellar signs and symptoms which subside, when the dose is reduced. Permanent cerebellar dysfunction has been suspected as a result of prolonged severe overdosage of phenytoin. A reversible acute cerebellar syndrome can occur with 5-fluorouracil.

Myelopathy

Myeloradiculopathy and arachnoid adhesions may rarely occur as a result of radiographic contrast media instilled into the subarachnoid space of the spinal cord for myelography.[2]

Neuromuscular Syndromes

Weakness of muscles due to myopathy with vacuolar and/or hyaline degeneration demonstrable in the biopsy material has been observed following treatment with fluorinated corticosteroids such as triamcinolone. This has occurred usually following prolonged treatment with high doses of severe rheumatoid arthritis or collagen disease. Prolonged treatment of rheumatoid arthritis with chloroquine may be complicated by a neuromyopathy affecting the pelvic girdle muscles. Tremors and muscle weakness are frequent signs of toxicity with lithium therapy. Muscle pain and stiffness are common after the use of succinylcholine, sometimes accompanied by myoglobinuria. Usual doses of succinylcholine may cause prolonged paralysis in individuals with atypical pseudocholinesterase who cannot metabolize succinylcholine rapidly enough. Profound muscle weakness and muscle damage can be caused by carbenoxolone, if severe hypokalemia is allowed to develop.

The polymyxin and aminoglycoside antibiotics can lead to neuromuscular blockade culminating in respiratory paralysis, particularly if high doses are used or in the presence of impaired renal function.[5] The clinical picture resembles the signs and symptoms of myasthenia gravis which can usually be reversed by neostigmine or calcium in the case of aminoglycosides. Withdrawal of the antibiotic is necessary in the case of polymyxins. As already discussed in a previous section, these agents should therefore be used with great care in patients with myasthenia gravis. Similarly, caution is in order when they are used in conjunction with skeletal muscle relaxants in bowel surgery. Muscle weakness and myasthenic signs have been noted in patients treated with penicillamine for rheumatoid arthritis or Wilson's disease.

Peripheral Neuropathy

Peripheral neuropathy has been caused by a variety of drugs. Clinically it may be manifested either by motor or sensory loss or both. Among the drugs that can cause neuropathy are antimicrobial agents such as nitrofurantoin, chloramphenicol, sulfonamides, kanamycin, streptomycin, polymyxin B, colistin and isoniazid.[6] In the case of the latter, the mechanism probably involves the induced pyridoxine deficiency which is most likely to occur in the slow isoniazid inactivators. Further drugs which can cause peripheral neuropathy include vincristine,[8] monoamine oxidase inhibitors, tricyclic antidepressants, chloroquine, disulfiram, arsenicals, emetine, procarbazine, and phenytoin.

The onset of drug-induced peripheral neuropathy may be heralded by paresthesias and dysesthesias and patients with these complaints should always be examined for other evidence of neuropathy such as sensory losses, subtle weakness and changes in the deep tendon reflexes. If the paresthesias are severe and persistent, it is probably best to stop the suspected drug, if possible. It is essential to stop nitrofurantoin and any other drug which can cause severe neuropathy.

REFERENCES

1. DE JONG R: Neurological complications of drugs with primary action on the nervous system. NY State J Med 70: 1857–1859, 1970.
2. HOLLISTER LE: Disorders of nervous system due to drugs. In: Drug Induced Diseases. (eds) Meyler OD, Peck CT. Excerpta Medica, Amsterdam, pp. 549–563, 1972.
3. JAMES IM: Diseases affecting drug responses. B & J Hosp Med 12: 823–831, 1974.
4. McQUILLEN MP: Hazards from antibiotics in myasthenia gravis. Ann Int Med 73: 487–496, 1970.
5. RICHET G, DE NOVALES, EL, VERROUST P: Drug intoxication and neurological episodes in chronic renal failure. Br Med J 2: 394–396, 1970.
6. ROBSON JM, SULLIVAN FM: Antituberculosis drugs. Pharmacol Rev 15: 169–223, 1963.
7. RUSSELL AS, LINDSTROM JM: Penicillamine-induced myasthenia gravis associated with antibodies to acetylcholine receptor. Neurology 28: 847–849, 1978.
8. WEISS HD, WALKER MD, WIERNIK PH: Neurotoxicity of commonly used antineoplastic agents. N Engl J Med 291: 75–78, 1974.

Index

Page numbers followed by (*t*) represent tables.

Abscess
   brain. *See* Brain abscess
   spinal epidural, 183–184
Acetazolamide, as antiepileptic drug,
   45
Acetylcholine (AcCh)
   drugs antagonistic to, 57
   in myasthenia gravis, 93, 94, 98
   in pseudomyasthenia (Lambert-
      Eaton syndrome), 99
   receptor substance (AcChR) in
      myasthenia gravis, 93, 97
Acetylsalicylic acid, in treatment of
      transient cerebral ischemic at-
      tack, 81
ACTH. *See* Corticotrophin (ACTH)
Actinomyces israelii, meningitis by,
      172
Addisonian pernicious anemia and
      cyanocobalamin (vitamin
      B-12) deficiency, 130
Adenine arabinoside (ARA-A,
      vidarabine), in treatment of
      Herpes simplex encephalitis,
      156, 184

Adrenal cortical insufficiency, 118
Adrenaline, 192
Adrenocorticotrophic hormone. *See*
      Corticotrophin (ACTH)
Akathisia, 191
Alcohol
   peripheral neuropathy, 122–123
   toxic delirium caused by, 190
   vitamin deficiencies and, 127
Alpha methyldopa
   in treatment of
      hypertensive encephalopathy, 87
      primary intracerebral hemor-
         rhage, 86
      subarachnoidal hemorrhage, 84
   toxic delirium caused by, 190
Alpha-methyl-dopa hydrazine (car-
      bidopa), 58, 59, 61, 67
Amantadine hydrochloride, in treat-
      ment of Parkinson's disease,
      65
Ambenonium, in treatment of myas-
      thenia gravis, 94, 95
Amebiasis, 172–173

Amikacin, in treatment of meningitis by
    gram-negative bacilli, 166–167
γ-Aminobutyric acid, 55
    lowered in Huntington's chorea, 69
ε-Aminocaproic acid, in treatment of
        subarachnoidal hemorrhage,
        84–85
Aminoglycosides, 141, 151, 161, 193
    adverse effects in myasthenia
        gravis, 189
    in treatment of
        infections of the central nervous
            system, 151
        meningitis, 165
        meningitis by gram-negative
            bacilli, 166, 167
        meningitis by *Listeria*
            monocytogenes, 165
        meningitis suspected, 174, 175
        spinal epidural abscess, 183
    penetration of cerebrospinal fluid
        (CSF), 137
Amitriptyline, in treatment of post-
        herpetic neuralgias, 112
Amobarbital, as antiepileptic drug, 48
Amphetamines, convulsions by, 190
Amphotericin B, in treatment of brain
        abscess, 181
    infections of the central nervous
        system, 152–154
    meningitis, 171–172, 173
    meningitis suspected, 174, 176
Ampicillin, 151, 161
    in treatment of
        brain abscess, 180, 181
        infections of the central nervous
            system, 149
        meningitis, 165
        meningitis by gram-negative
            bacilli, 166, 167
        meningitis by *Haemophilus in-*
            fluenzae, 165–166

meningitis by *Listeria*
    monocytogenes, 164–165
meningitis suspected, 174–177
streptococcal and neisserian
    meningitis, 158
sensitivity of *Escherichia coli* to,
    137
Analgesics, in treatment of
    postherpetic neuralgias, 112
    trigeminal neuralgia, 111
Anemia
    Addisonian pernicious, and
        cyanocobalamin (vitamin
        B-12) deficiency, 130
    megaloblastic, and cyanocobala-
        min (vitamin B-12) deficiency,
        129–130
    megaloblastic, and folic acid defi-
        ciency, 131
Antianxiety drugs, toxic delirium by,
    190
Antibacterial agents commonly used
        in infections of the central ner-
        vous system, 147–152
Antibiotics, adverse effects in myas-
        thenia gravis of, 189
Anticholinergic agents
    in treatment of Parkinson's disease,
        57–58, 58t, 72
    toxic delirium caused by, 190
Anticholinesterase, in treatment of
        myasthenia gravis, 94–95, 98
Anticoagulants, in treatment of
    cerebral emboli, 83
    progressing stroke, 82
    transient cerebral ischemic attack,
        80–81
Anticonvulsant therapy, 142–143
Antidepressants, toxic delirium by
    tricyclic, 190
Antiepileptic drugs, 17–38, 38t
    dose and blood level relations, 40t
    historical notes, 17–18

Antifungal agents commonly used for infections of the central nervous system, 152–155
Antihistamines, 191
Antimicrobial agents
  important adverse reactions, 140–141*t*
  in treatment of brain abscess, 179
  relative penetration into the central nervous system, 138*t*
  therapy for central nervous system infection of known etiology, 162–163*t*
Antiparkinsonian drugs, 191
Antipsychotic drugs, toxic delirium by, 190
Antisera and brain syndromes, 192
Antituberculous agents commonly used for infections of the central nervous system, 155–156
Antiviral agents commonly used for infections of the central nervous system, 156
Apomorphine, in treatment of Parkinson's disease, 56, 63, 65
ARA-A (adenine arabinoside, vidarabine), 156, 184
Arteritis, temporal, 87–88
Arthritis, rheumatoid, and neuromuscular syndromes, 193
1-Asparaginase, and encephalopathy, 192
Aspirin, in treatment of transient cerebral ischemic attack, 81
Atherosclerosis and cerebrovascular diseases, 76–78
Atropine, in treatment of myasthenia gravis, 94, 98

Baclofen, in treatment of spasticity in multiple sclerosis, 103–104
Bacterial meningitis. *See* Meningitis: bacterial

Barbiturates
  adverse effects in migraine, 189–190
  as antiepileptic drugs, 48
  in treatment of
    acute migraine attack, 107
    hemiballismus, 68
    Sydenham's (infectious) chorea, 70
  preventive therapy of migrainous headaches, 110
BCNU (1,3-bis(2-chloroethyl)-1-nitrosourea), in treatment of malignant gliomas, 134–135
Bemegride, convulsions by, 190
Benserazide, in treatment of Parkinson's disease, 61
Benzodiazepines
  as antiepileptic drugs, 45, 47
  preventive therapy for migrainous headaches, 110
Benztropine mesylate, in treatment of Parkinson's disease, 57, 72
Benzyl penicillin, in treatment of infections of the central nervous system, 148–149
Beriberi and thiamine deficiency, 129
Bicarbonate, in treatment of diabetic coma with acidosis, 115
Biguanidines, in treatment of diabetic peripheral neuropathy, 122
1,3-Bis(2-chloroethyl)-1-nitrosourea (BCNU), in treatment of malignant gliomas, 134–135
Blood levels of drugs in nervous system disorders, 7–8
Brain
  abscess, 177–182
    antimicrobial therapy, 160*t*
    diagnosis, 178
    general considerations, 177–178
    management, 178–182

Brain (*continued*)
  management: anticonvulsant
    therapy, 182
  management: antimicrobial
    therapy, 179–182
  management: debridement of
    continguous foci, 181–182
  management: definitive anti-
    biotic regimen, 181
  management: initial antimicro-
    bial therapy, 180–181
  management: long term, 182
  management: medical decom-
    pression, 179
  athetosis, 66–67
  circulation, drug-induced compli-
    cations related to, 192
  edema
    agents to try to reduce, 82
    medical management, 142
  infarction, 78–79, 82–83
  injury and tumor predisposing to
    seizure disorders, 12–13
  ischemia, 78–81
Bromocriptine, in treatment of Parkinson's disease, 63, 65
Butyrophenones, 191

Caffeine, absorption of ergotamine
  tartrate facilitated by, 107
Calciferol, in treatment of hypocalcemia, 119
Calcitonin, 119
Calcium, in treatment of hypocalcemia, 119
Candida infections, treatment with
  5-fluorocytosine (5-FC) of, 154
Carbamazepine
  as antiepileptic drug, 18–20, 44–45
  in treatment of trigeminal neuralgia,
    111

Carbenicillin
  in treatment of
    brain abscess, 181
    infections of the central nervous
      system, 150
    meningitis by gram-negative
      bacilli, 166, 167
    meningitis suspected, 176
  sensitivity of *Pseudomonas* to, 139
Carbidopa (alpha methyl-dopa hydrazine), 58, 59
Carbon dioxide, inhalation to produce cerebral vasodilation, 82
Cardiac dysrhythmia, 78
Catecholamines, extrapyramidal syndromes by agents blocking
  brain, 191
CCNU (1-(2-chloroethyl)-3-
  cyclohexyl-nitrosourea, in
  treatment of malignant
  gliomas, 134–135
Central nervous system infections.
  See Infections of the central
  nervous system
Cephaloridine, in treatment of
  staphylococcal meningitis,
  161
Cephalosporins
  contraindications for
    meningitis by *Staphylococcus*,
      161
    meningitis by *Streptococcus* and
      Neisssria, 158
  in treatment of
    infections of the central nervous
      system, 150
    tetanus, 185
  penetration of cerebrospinal fluid
    (CSF), 137
Cephalothin, in treatment of
  brain abscess, 180
  meningitis by *Staphylococcus*, 161

Cerebellar syndromes, drug-induced, 192
Cerebrospinal fluid (CSF) in meningitis, 157–158
Cerebrospinal shunts or reservoirs, infection of, 167–168
Cerebrovascular diseases, 76–88
  cerebral emboli, 83
  hypertensive encephalopathy, 87
  introduction and general principles, 76–78
  predisposing to seizure disorders, 13
  primary intracerebral hemorrhage, 85–87
  progressing stroke, 78, 81–83
  subarachnoidal hemorrhage, 84–85
  teporal arteritis, 87–88
  transient ischemic attack, 78–81
  transient ischemic attack and stroke, 81
Chlamydia, infections by, 173
Chloramphenicol, 141, 151, 152
  in treatment of
    brain abscess, 180, 181
    infections of the central nervous system, 147–148
    meningitis by *Clostridium*, 164
    meningitis by gram-negative bacilli, 166–167
    meningitis by *Haemophilus influenzae*, 165–166
    meningitis by *Listeria monocytogenes*, 164–165
    meningitis by *Pseudomonas*, 166
    meningitis by *Staphylococcus*, 161, 164
    meningitis by *Streptococcus* and *Neisseria*, 158
    meningitis suspected, 174–177
    rickettsial diseases, 185
    tularemia, 185
    sensitivity of *Escherichia coli* to, 137
Chlordiazepoxide, in treatment of postherpetic neuralgias, 112
Chlormethiazole, as antiepileptic drug, 48
1-(2-Chloroethyl)-3-cyclohexyl-nitrosourea (CCNU), in treatment of malignant gliomas, 134–135
1-(2-Chloroethyl)-3-(4-methylcyclohexyl)-1-nitrosourea (Me CCNU), in treatment of malignant gliomas, 134–135
Chloroquine
  in treatment of
    meningitis by *Entamoeba histolytica*, 173
    rheumatoid arthritis, neuromuscular syndromes in, 193
    resistance to in meningitis by malaria, 172
Chlorpromazine, in treatment of
  hemiballismus, 68
  postherpetic neuralgias, 112
  Sydenham's (infectious) chorea, 70
Chorea
  Huntington's, 68–69
  Sydenham's (infectious), 69–70
Clindamycin
  contraindications for meningitis by *Staphylococcus*, 161
    Streptococcus and *Neisseria*, 158
  in treatment of infections of the central nervous system, 152
  penetration of cerebrospinal fluid (CSF), 137
Clonazepam, as antiepileptic drug, 20–21, 47
Clostridium, meningitis by, 164
Clostridium tetani infections, 185

Clotrimazole, contraindicated in infections of the central nervous system, 155
Codeine, in treatment of
  acute migraine attack, 107, 108
  postherpetic neuralgias, 112
Colistin, adverse effects in myasthenia gravis of, 189
Coma
  diabetic, with ketoacidosis, 115
  hyperosmotic, 116
  hypoosmotic, 116–117
Contraceptive agents, oral
  and brain syndromes, 192
  and cerebral circulation, 192
  preventive therapy for migrainous headaches, 110
Convulsions, drug-induced, 190–191
Copper, abnormalities due to, in hepatolenticular degeneration (Wilson's disease), 65–66
Corticosteroids
  and encephalopathy, 192
  and neuromuscular syndromes, 193
  in treatment of
    cerebral edema, 142
    fungal meningitis, 171
    malignant gliomas, 133–134
    multiple sclerosis, 102
    Sydenham's (infectious) chorea, 70
    tuberculous meningitis, 170
Corticotrophin (ACTH), 47
  diagnosis of hypoadrenalism, 118
  in treatment of
    hypoadrenalism, 118
    multiple sclerosis, 102
    myasthenia gravis, 95, 96
Cortisol, in treatment of hypothyroid encephalopathy, 118
Co-trimoxazole, 150–151

Coumadin, as anticoagulant in
  cerebral emboli, 83
  progressing stroke, 82
  transient cerebral ischemic attack, 80, 82
Cryptococcus, meningitis suspected by, 174, 176
Curare, in treatment of tetanus, 185
Curare-like agents, in treatment of myasthenic crises, 98
Cyanocobalamin (vitamin B-12), 128
  deficiency, 129–130
Cycloserine
  convulsions caused by, 191
  in treatment of tuberculous meningitis, 169
Cyproheptadine, in preventive therapy for migrainous headaches, 108, 109
Cytosine arabinoside (ARA-C), contraindications for viral encephalitis, 184

Dantrolene, in treatment of spasticity in multiple sclerosis, 103, 104
Decadron, in treatment of cerebral edema, 142
Decarboxylase inhibitor, 56, 58–64, 67, 71
  in treatment of Parkinson's disease with levodopa and, 60t
Degenerative nervous system diseases little affected by current chemotherapeutic agents, 2
Delirium, drug-induced toxic, 190
Dementia in Parkinson's disease, 64
Demyelination in multiple sclerosis, 101
Dexamethasone, in treatment of brain abscess, 179
  malignant gliomas, 135
Dextrose solution, in treatment of

diabetic coma with acidosis, 115

Diabetes insipidus
  hyperosmotic coma in, 116
  hypoosmotic coma in, 116–117

Diabetes mellitus
  coma with ketoacidosis, 115
  hyperosmotic coma in, 116
  hypoglycemia, 116
  peripheral neuropathy, 121–122

Diazepam, in treatment of
  convulsions, 143, 182
  dystonia musculorum deformans, 68
  epilepsy, 21–23, 44, 47, 48
  overdose of ergotamine or dihydroergotamine, 108
  postherpetic neuralgias, 112
  spasticity in multiple sclerosis, 103
  tetanus, 185

Diazoxide, in treatment of hypertensive encephalopathy, 87

Digitalis, toxic delirium by, 190

Dihydroergotamine mesylate, 108

Dihydroxyphenylalanine. *See* Dopa

Dimethadione (DMO), as product of trimethadione (TMO) metabolism, 46

Diphenhydramine, in treatment of drug-induced Parkinson's disease, 72

Dipyridamole, in treatment of transient cerebral ischemic attack, 81

Diuretic agents
  and encephalopathy, 192
  osmotic, in treatment of
    brain abscess, 179
    brain edema, 142

Dopa (dihydroxyphenylalanine), 56–57, 59, 61–64

in diagnosing Huntington's chorea, 69

Dopamine, 55–56, 69

Doxepin, in treatment of postherpetic neuralgias, 112

Drug-induced
  dyskinesia, 71–72
  encephalopathy, 120–121
  extrapyramidal disorder, 71

Drugs, interaction between, 8–10
  biotransformation involved, 9
  drug absorption, 9
  drug distribution involved, 9–10
  occurring at site of action, 10

Drugs used in treatment of movement disorders, 67t

Dyskinesia, 191
  drug-induced, 71–72

Dysrhythmia, cardiac, 78

Dystonia musculorum deformans, 68
  torticollis, 68

Edema, brain
  agents to reduce, 82
  medical management, 142

Edrophonium, as diagnostic aid in myasthenia gravis, 94, 95

Emboli, cerebral, 83

Emetine, in treatment of meningitis by *Entamoeba histolytica*, 173

Empyema, subdural, 182–183

Encephalitis, 156, 184

Encephalopathy
  drug-induced, 120–121, 192
  liver, 117
  metabolic
    congenital enzyme deficiencies, 119–120
    diabetic coma with ketoacidosis, 115
    diabetic hypoglycemia, 116
    hyperosmotic coma, 116

Encephalopathy (*continued*)
    hypoadrenalism, 118
    hypocalcemia, 119
    hypoosmotic coma, 116–117
    hypothyroid, 118
    phenylketonuria, 119–120
Entamoeba histolytica, meningitis by,
    172–173
Enzyme deficiencies, congenital,
    119–120
Epilepsies and pregnancy, 20, 24, 27,
    32–33, 35, 37–38, 49–50
Epilepsies, treatment of
  absence (petit mal) seizures, 45–47
  basic considerations, 38–39
  blood level of drugs, 39–41
    how to store samples, 41
    plasma versus serum, 41
    units in laboratory reports, 41
    what blood levels to order, 41
    when to draw blood, 41
    when to order, 40
  clinical considerations, 41–42
  drug dose and blood level relations,
    40*t*
  drugs. *See* Antiepileptic drugs
  myoclonic seizures, 47
  partial complex (temporal lobe)
    seizures, 44–45
  precautions, 42–43
  status epilepticus, 47–49
  tonic-clonic seizures (primary or
    secondary grand mal), 43–44
  when to start therapy, 42
Epileptics, birth defects in general
    population and, 32*t*
Epsilon aminocaproic acid, in treat-
    ment of subarachnoidal
    hemorrhage, 84–85
Ergot derivatives, in treatment of Par-
    kinson's disease, 56, 65

Ergotamine tartrate
  in treatment of
    acute migraine attack, 106–108
    cluster headaches (migraine
      neuralgia), 110
  side effects, 108
Erythromycin, in treatment of
  infections of the central nervous
    system, 151
  meningitis by *Listeria*
    monocytogenes, 165
  meningitis by *Staphylococcus*, 161
  meningitis by *Streptococcus* and
    Neisseria, 158
  Mycoplasma pneumoniae infec-
    tions, 173
Escherichia coli, meningitis by, 165,
    166
Essential tremor, 70
Ethambutol, in treatment of tuber-
    culosis, 155–156, 169–170
Ethionamide, in treatment of tuber-
    culous meningitis, 169
Ethosuximide, as antiepileptic drug,
    23–24, 45–47
Extrapyramidal syndromes, 54–72
  cerebral athetosis, 66–67
  drug-induced, 71, 191
    dyskinesia, 71–72
    extrapyramidal disorder, 71
  dystonia musculorum deformans,
    68
    torticollis, 68
  essential tremor, 70
  hemiballismus, 67–68
  hepatolenticular degeneration
    (Wilson's disease), 65–66
  Huntington's chorea, 68–69
  Parkinson's disease, 54–65
  Sydenham's (infectious) chorea,
    69–70

Facial pain. *See* Head pain: facial
     pain
Flurazepam, in treatment of acute mi-
     graine attack, 107
5-Fluorocytosine (5-FC), 152, 171–
     172
  in treatment of central nervous sys-
     tem infections, 154
5-Fluorouracil, and cerebellar syn-
     dromes, 152
Folic acid
  deficiency, 131
  to reduce birth defects, 49
Fungal meningitis, 170–172

Gamma-aminobutyric acid, 55
  lowered in Huntington's chorea, 69
Genetic factors predisposing to sei-
     zure disorders, 13
Gentamicin
  adverse effects in myasthenia
     gravis, 189
  in treatment of
     brain abscess, 181
     infections of the central nervous
     system, 151
     meningitis by *Escherichia coli*,
     165
     meningitis by gram-negative
     bacilli, 166
     meningitis suspected, 174, 176
  sensitivity to, of
     Escherichia coli, 137
     Pseudomonas, 139
Gliomas, malignant
  postoperative therapy of, 134*t*
  treatment of, 133–135
Glucagon, in treatment of diabetic
     hypoglycemia, 116
Glucocorticosteroids, in treatment of
     brain abscess, 179, 182

Glucose, in treatment of diabetic
     hypoglycemia, 116
Glutamic acid decarboxylase, low-
     ered in Huntington's chorea,
     69
Glutethimide, in treatment of essential
     tremor, 70
Glycerol
  in treatment of
     brain abscess, 179
     brain edema, 142
  to produce brain vasodilation, 82
Gonococcus, meningitis by, 164
Guanidine, in treatment of
     pseudomyasthenia (Lambert-
     Eaton syndrome), 99

Haemophilus influenzae
  meningitis by, 165–166
  meningitis suspected by, 174
Haloperidol, 191
  in drug-induced Parkinson's dis-
     ease, 71
  in treatment of
     dystonia musculorum deformans,
     68
     Sydenham's (infectious) chorea,
     70
Head pain, 106–112
  facial pain, 110–112
     atypical, 112
     postherpetic neuralgias, 111–112
     trigeminal neuralgia, 111
  migrainous headaches, 106–110
     preventive therapy, 108–110
     treatment of acute attack, 106–
     108
     treatment of cluster headaches
     (migraine neuralgia), 110
Hemiballismus, 67–68

Hemorrhage
  primary intracerebral, 85–87
  subarachnoidal, 84–85
Heparin, as anticoagulant in progress-
    ing stroke, 82
Hepatic encephalopathy, 117
Hepatitis complicating antitubercul-
    ous therapy, 155, 156
Hepatolenticular degeneration (Wil-
    son's disease), 65–66
Hereditary nervous system diseases
  little affected by current
    chemotherapeutic agents, 2
Herpes simplex encephalitis,
    vidarabine (adenine
    arabinoside, ARA-A)
  treatment of, 156
Herpes zoster infection, neuralgias
    following, 111–112
Hexamethonium, 192
Huntington's chorea, 68–69
Hydrocephalus complicating brain
    abscess, 182
Hydrochlorothiazide, in treatment of
  periodic hypokalemic paralysis,
    124
Hydrocortisone, 154
  in treatment of hypoadrenalism,
    118
2-Hydroxystilbamidine, contraindica-
    tion for central nervous system
    infections of, 155
Hyperosmotic coma, 116
Hypertensive encephalopathy, 87
Hypoadrenalism, 118
Hypocalcemia, 119
Hypokalemic paralysis, periodic,
    123–124
Hypoosmotic coma, 116–117
Hypotension, orthostatic, accom-
    panying dihydroxyphenyl-

    alanine (dopa) therapy in
    Parkinson's disease, 61
Hypothyroid encephalopathy, 118

Idoxuridine (IUDR), contraindication
    for viral encephalitis of, 184
Imipramine, in treatment of post-
    herpetic neuralgias, 112
Immune globulin, tetanus, 185
Indomethacin, vertigo caused by, 192
Infarction, cerebral, 78–79, 82–83
Infections of the central nervous sys-
    tem, 136–185
  antibacterial agents commonly
    used, 147–152
  anticonvulsant therapy, 142–143
  antifungal agents commonly used,
    152–155
  antimicrobial therapy when etiol-
    ogy known, 162–163*t*
  antituberculous agents commonly
    used, 155–156
  antiviral agents commonly used,
    156
  choice of antimicrobial regimen,
    137–139
  complications, 143, 147, 147*t*
  conditions predisposing to, 143,
    144–146*t*
  medical management of cerebral
    edema, 142
  predisposing to seizure disorders,
    13
  specified microbial diagnosis, 139,
    141
  surgical management, 141–142
Infectious (Sydenham's) chorea,
    69–70
Insulin
  as cause of diabetic hypoglycemia,
    116

in treatment of
    diabetic coma with acidosis, 115
    diabetic peripheral neuropathy,
      122
International League Against Epilepsy
    Classification of Seizures, 15*t*
Iodides, contraction for infections of
      the central nervous system of,
      155
Ischemia, brain, 78–81
    and stroke, 81
Isoniazid (INH)
    convulsions as adverse effects of,
      191
    in treatment of tuberculosis, 155,
      169–170
    pharmacogenetic factors, 6
    pyridoxine action antagonized by,
      131

Kanamycin
    adverse effects in myasthenia
      gravis, 189
    in treatment of meningitis, 165
    by gram-negative bacilli, 166
Klebsiella, meningitis by, 165
Korsakoff's psychosis and thiamine
      deficiency, 129

Lactulose, in treatment of hepatic en-
      cephalopathy, 117
Lambert-Eaton syndrome
      (pseudomyasthenia), 99
Leptospirosis, 168–169
Lergotril mesylate, in treatment of
      Parkinson's disease, 65
Levodopa
    diagnosis of Huntington's chorea,
      69
    in treatment of
      cerebral athetosis, 67

      Parkinson's disease, 58–59, 60*t*,
        61, 64, 71
Lidocaine, convulsions as adverse
      reaction to, 191
Lincomycin, in treatment of infections
      of the central nervous system,
      152
Listeria monocytogenes, meningitis
      by, 164–165
Lithium, toxicity with neuromuscular
      syndromes, 193
Lithium carbonate, and brain syn-
      dromes, 192
Liver encephalopathy, 117

Malaria, 172
Malignant gliomas
    postoperative therapy of, 134*t*
    treatment of, 133–135
Mannitol, in treatment of
    brain abscess, 179
    brain edema, 142
Me CCNU (1-(2-chloroethyl)-3-
      (4-methylcyclohexyl)-1-nitro-
      sourea), in treatment of malig-
      nant gliomas, 134–135
Megaloblastic anemia
    and cyanocobalamin (vitamin
      B-12) deficiency, 129–130
    and folic acid deficiency, 131
Melarsoprol, in treatment of en-
      cephalitis associated with
      trypanosomiasis, 173
Meningitis
    Actinomyces israelii, 172
    antimicrobial therapy, 159*t*
    bacterial
      gram-negative bacilli, 165–167
      gram-positive and gram-negative
        cocci, 158, 161, 164
      gram-positive bacilli, 164–165

Meningitis (*continued*)
 multiple organisms, 167
 fungal, 170–172
 general considerations, 156–158
 microbial
  partially-treated bacterial, 176–177
  suspected but not immediately documented, 173–177
  suspected in immunologically normal patients, 174–175
  suspected in patients with known predisposition to, 175–176
 Nocardia asteroides, 172
 parasitic
  helminthic, 173
  protozoan, 172–173
 spirochaetal, 168–169
 staphylococcal, 161, 164
 tuberculous, 169–170
 viral, 169
  suspected, 175
Mephenytoin, as antiepileptic drug, 24–25
Meprobamate, in treatment of tetanus, 185
Metabolic encephalopathy. *See* Encephalopathy: metabolic
Methicillin, in treatment of
 infections of the central nervous system, 149–150
 meningitis by *Staphylococcus*, 161
Methotrexate, and encephalopathy, 192
Methsuximide, as antiepileptic drug, 45
α-Methyldopa
 in treatment of
  hypertensive encephalopathy, 87
  primary intracerebral hemorrhage, 86

subarachnoidal hemorrhage, 84
 toxic delirium caused by, 190
α-Methyl-dopa hydrazine (carbidopa), 58, 59, 61, 67
Methylmalonyl Co-A, conversion to succinyl Co-A, 130
Methyl orednisolone, in treatment of brain edema, 142
Methysergide
 in treatment of cluster headaches (migraine neuralgia), 110
 preventive therapy for migrainous headaches, 108–109
Metoclopramide, 191
Metronidazole, in treatment of meningitis by *Entamoeba histolytica*, 173
Miconazole, 171
 in treatment of infections of the central nervous system, 154–155
Migraine, drug-induced, 189
Migrainous headaches. *See* Head pain: migrainous headaches
Monoamine oxidase inhibitors, 192
Monoamine transmitters and migrainous headaches, 106
Movement disorders, drugs used in treatment of, 67*t*
Multiple sclerosis, 101–104
 agents tried and failed, 101
 spasticity, 103–104
 steroid treatment, 102–103
Myasthenia gravis, 92–99
 anticholinesterase therapy, 94–95
 crises and treatment of crises, 97–98
 drug-induced worsening, 189
 immunosuppressive chemotherapy, 95–97
 in newborns, 97
 pathophysiology, 92–93

pseudomyasthenia (Lambert-Eaton syndrome), 99
therapy, 93–98
Mycoplasma pneumoniae, infections by, 173
Myelopathy, drug-induced, 193
Myopathies, 123–124
Myxedema, 118

Nafcillin, in treatment of
brain abscess, 181
infections of the central nervous system, 149–150
meningitis by *Staphylococcus*, 161, 164
meningitis suspected, 175, 176
spinal epidural abscess, 183
Nalidixic acid
brain syndromes, 192
convulsions caused by, 191
Neisseria gonorrhoeae, meningitis by, 164
Neisseria meningitidis, meningitis by, 158
Neomycin, in treatment of
hepatic encephalopathy, 117
myasthenic crises, 98
Neostigmine, 193
in treatment of myasthenia gravis, 94, 95, 98
Nervous system complications with systemic metabolic disorders, 114–124
Nervous system disorders
degenerative and/or hereditary, little affected by current chemotherapeutic agents, 2
drug-induced, 189–194
drug therapy, 1–10
blood levels, 7–8

interactions between drugs, 8–10
pharmacodynamic aspects, 2–3, 8
pharmacogenetic aspects, 6–7
pharmacokinetic aspects, 3–8
Nervous system infections. *See* Infections of the central nervous system
Neuralgia
migraine, 110
postherpetic, 111–112
trigeminal, 111
Neuromuscular disorders, drug-induced, 189, 193
Neuropathy, peripheral
alcoholic, 122–123
diabetic, 121–122
drug-induced, 193–194
Newborns, myasthenia gravis in, 97
Niacin (nicotinic acid), deficiency of, 128
Nitrosoureas, in treatment of malignant gliomas, 133–135
Nocardia asteroides, meningitis by, 172
Noradrenaline, 55, 192

Opiates, 190, 192
Oral contraceptives
and brain circulation, 192
and brain syndromes, 192
preventive therapy of migrainous headaches, 110
Orthostatic hypotension accompanying dihydroxyphenylalanine (dopa) therapy in Parkinson's disease, 61
Osmotic diuretics, in treatment of
brain abscess, 179
brain edema, 142

Oxacillin, in treatment of
  infections of the central nervous
      system, 149–150
  meningitis by *Staphylococcus*, 161
  spinal epidural abscess, 183

Pain, head. *See* Head pain
Papaverine, to produce brain vasodi-
      lation, 82
Paracetamol, in treatment of acute
      migraine attack, 106
Paralysis, periodic hypokalemic,
      123–124
Parasitic meningitis, 172–173
Parkinson's disease
  abnormal involuntary movements a
      side effect of drug therapy,
      61–62
  dementia in, 64
  diagnosis, 54–55
  orthostatic hypotension accom-
      panying dihydroxyphenyl-
      alanine (dopa) therapy, 61
  pathophysiology, 55–56
  postural instability, 63
  treatment, 56–64
  treatment with levodopa and a de-
      carboxylase inhibitor, 60*t*
Pavulon, in treatment of tetanus, 185
Penicillamine, pyridoxine action an-
      tagonized by, 131
Penicillin, 141, 152
  in treatment of
      actinomycosis, 172
      brain abscess, 180
      meningitis, 164
      meningitis by *Actinomyces is-
          raelii*, 172
      meningitis by *Clostridium*, 164
      meningitis by gram-negative
          bacilli, 167

  meningitis by *Listeria
      monocytogenes*, 164–165
  meningitis suspected, 175, 176
Penicillin G
  aqueous crystalline (benzyl), 148–
      149
  convulsions as adverse effect, 190
  in treatment of
      meningitis by *Streptococcus* and
          Neisseria, 158
      meningitis suspected, 174
      syphilitic central nervous system
          infections, drug of choice for,
          168–169
      tetanus, 185
Penicillin, penicillinase resistant, in
      treatment of
  infections of the central nervous
      system, 149–150
  meningitis by *Staphylococcus*, 161
  meningitis suspected, 175
Pentazocine, in treatment of
  acute migraine attack, 107, 108
  postherpetic neuralgias, 112
Pentobarbital, in treatment of acute
      migraine attack, 107
Pentolinium, 192
Pernicious anemia (Addisonian) and
      cyanocobalamin (vitamin
      B-12) deficiency, 130
Pertussis vaccine and brain syn-
      dromes, 192
Pharmacodynamic aspects of treat-
      ment, 2–3, 8
Pharmacogenetic aspects of treat-
      ment, 6–7
Pharmacokinetic aspects of treatment,
      3–8
  absorption, 3–4
  biotransformation, 4–5
  distribution, 5–6

elimination, 4–5
plasma half-life, 4
Phenacetamide, as antiepileptic drug,
45
Phenobarbital (phenobarbitone)
conversion from primidone, 33–34
in treatment of
convulsions, 143
epilepsy, 25–27, 33, 44, 46, 48,
50
hemiballismus, 68
Sydenham's (infectious) chorea,
70
pharmacogenetic aspects, 6–7
Phenothiazines
extrapyramidal syndromes as adverse reactions, 191
in drug-induced Parkinson's disease, 71, 72
in treatment of
acute migraine attack, 107
dystonia musculorum deformans,
68
hemiballismus, 68
Huntington's chorea, 69
preventive therapy for migrainous
headaches, 110
Phensuximide, as antiepileptic drug,
45
Phenylalanine, in phenylketonuria,
119–120
Phenylethyl-malonamide (PEMA),
conversion from primidone of,
33–34
Phenytoin, 27–33, 43–44, 48, 50
as antiepileptic drug
administration and blood levels,
28–30
drugs that can cause changes of
blood level, 30*t*
formulation and indications,
27–28
in breast milk, 50
in pregnancy, 32–33, 32*t*
in treatment of convulsions, 141
interactions, 30–31, 30*t*
mechanism of action, 28
names (chemical and proprietary), 27
partial complex (temporal lobe)
seizures, 44
pharmacokinetic parameters, 28
relevant side effects, 31–32
status epilepticus, 48–49
tonic-clonic seizures (primary or
secondary grand mal), 43–44
cerebellar syndromes as adverse
reaction, 192
in treatment of
brain abscess, 182
trigeminal neuralgia, 111
pharmacogenetic factors, 6–7
relationship with folic acid deficiency, 131
Physostigmine, in treatment of myasthenia gravis, 94
Pimozide, 191
in treatment of Huntington's
chorea, 69
Piribedil (trivastal), in treatment of
Parkinson's disease, 56, 63, 65
Pisotifen, in preventive therapy for
migraine headaches, 108, 109
Plasmapheresis, in treatment of myasthenia gravis, 97
Plasmodium falciparum, meningitis
by, 172
Poliomyelitis, 184
Polymyxin, 193
Polymyxin B
adverse effects in myasthenia gravis
of, 189
in treatment of meningitis by
gram-negative bacilli, 166

Postherpetic neuralgias, 111–112
Postural instability in Parkinson's disease, 63
Potassium, in treatment of diabetic coma with acidosis, 115
Potassium chloride, in treatment of periodic hypokalemic paralysis, 123–124
Prednisone, in treatment of
    brain abscess, 179
    hypoadrenalism, 118
    multiple sclerosis, 102
    myasthenia gravis, 95–97
    Sydenham's (infectious) chorea, 70
    temporal arteritis, 88
Pregnancy and epilepsies, 20, 24, 27, 32–33, 35, 37–38, 49–50
Primidone
    as antiepileptic drug, 33–35, 44
    conversion to phenobarbital and phenylethyl-malonamide (PEMA), 33–34
Procaine, convulsions as adverse reaction to, 191
Procarbazine, to support nitrosoureas in treatment of malignant gliomas, 133–135
Prochlorperazine, in treatment of acute migraine attack, 107
Propoxyphene, in treatment of
    acute migraine attack, 106
    postherpetic neuralgias, 112
Propranolol, in treatment of
    essential tremor, 70
    migrainous headaches, 108, 109–110
Protein, restriction in diet for hepatic encephalopathy, 117
Pseudomonas, meningitis by, 165
Pseudomyasthenia (Lambert-Eaton syndrome), 99
Psychosis and thiamine deficiency, Korsakoff's, 129

Pyridostigmine, in treatment of myasthenia gravis, 94, 95, 98
Pyridoxine (vitamin B-6)
    deficiency, 131, 191
    in treatment of
        meningitis associated with toxoplasmosis, 173
        neuropathy during antituberculous therapy, 155

Quinidine, as cause of myasthenic crises, 98
Quinine, as cause of myasthenic crises, 98
Quinine dihydrochloride, in treatment of meningitis by malaria, 172

Rabies, 184
Rat bite fever, 168–169
Relapsing fever, 168–169
Reserpine
    in drug-induced Parkinson's disease, 71
    in treatment of
        Huntington's chorea, 69
        hypertensive encephalopathy, 87
        Parkinson's disease, 55
        primary intracerebral hemorrhage, 86
        subarachnoidal hemorrhage, 84
    toxic delirium by, 190
Rheumatoid arthritis and neuromuscular syndromes, 193
Rickettsia, infections by, 173, 185
Rifampin, in treatment of tuberculosis, 156, 169–170

Salicylates, in treatment of acute migraine attack, 106
Sclerosis, multiple, 101–104
    spasticity, 103–104
    steroid treatment, 102–103

Sedatives
  contraindication in hepatic en-
    cephalopathy, 117
  toxic delirium by, 190
Seizure disorders, 12–50
  classification, 14–17
    generalized seizures, 15–16
    partial seizures, 16
    unclassified seizures, 16–17
    unilateral seizures, 16
  International League Against
    Epilepsy
  Classification of Seizures, 15*t*
  predisposing factors
    brain tumor, 12–13
    cerebrovascular disease, 13
    genetic factors, 13
    head and brain injury, 12
    infections, 13
    process, 13–14
    types, 14
Serotonin, 55
  and migrainous headaches, 106–
    108
  antagonists in preventive therapy of
    migrainous headaches, 108,
    109
  brain, extrapyramidal syndromes
    by agents blocking, 191
Serum glutamic oxalacetic trans-
    aminase (SGOT), 37, 43, 46,
    63, 135
Serum glutamic pyruvic transaminase
    (SGPT), 37, 43, 46, 135
Smallpox vaccine and brain syn-
    dromes, 192
Sodium, in treatment of hypoosmotic
    coma, 117
Sodium nitroprusside, in treatment of
  hypertensive encephalopathy, 87
  primary intracerebral hemorrhage,
    86

Spinal cord degeneration and
    cyanocobalamin (vitamin
    B-12) deficiency, 129
Spinal epidural abscess, 183–184
Spirochaetal meningitis, 168–169
Staphylococcus aureus, meningitis
    by, 161, 164
Staphylococcus epidermidis, menin-
    gitis by, 161, 164
Steroid hormones, in treatment of
    Sydenham's (infectious)
    chorea, 70
Steroids, in treatment of
  brain abscess, 179
  temporal arteritis, 88
  underlying conditions with brain
    emboli, 83
Streptococcus pneumoniae, menin-
    gitis by, 158, 164
Streptomycin
  in treatment of
    tuberculous meningitis, 170
    tularemia, 185
  myasthenia gravis as adverse effect,
    189
Stroke, progressing, 78, 81–83
Subdural empyema, 182–183
Succinylcholine, 193
Succinyl Co-A, conversion from
    methylmalonyl Co-A of, 130
Sulfamethoxazole, 150–151, 173
Sulfinpyrazone, in treatment of trans-
    ient cerebral ischemic attack,
    81
Sulfonamides
  contraindications for in meningitis
    by *Streptococcus* and *Neis-
    seria*, 158
  in treatment of
    infections of the central nervous
      system, 150–151
    meningitis associated with toxo-
      plasmosis, 173

Sulfonamides (*continued*)
meningitis by *Nocardia asteroides*, 172
Sulfonylureas, in treatment of diabetic peripheral neuropathy, 122
Suramin, in treatment of encephalitis associated with trypanosomiasis, 173
Sydenham's (infectious) chorea, 69–70
Sympathomimetic drugs, 192
Syphilis, 168–169

Temporal arteritis, 87–88
Tetanus, 185
antitoxin and brain syndromes, 192
Tetrabenazine, 191
in drug-induced Parkinson's disease, 71
in treatment of
dystonia musculorum deformans, 68
Huntington's chorea, 69
Tetracycline
and brain syndromes, 192
contraindications for in meningitis by *Streptococcus* and *Neisseria*, 158
in treatment of
infections of the central nervous system, 152
Mycoplasma pneumoniae infections, 173
rickettsial diseases, 185
tetanus, 185
tularemia, 185
Thiamine, deficiency of, 129
Thiethylperazine, in treatment of acute migraine attack, 107
Thiothixene, 191
Thioxanthenes, 191
Thymectomy, in treatment of myasthenia gravis, 96, 97

Thyroid hormones, in treatment of hypothyroid encephalopathy, 118
Thyroxine, in treatment of hypothyroid encephalopathy, 118
Ticarcillin, in treatment of infections of the central nervous system, 150
Tobramycin, in treatment of
infections of the central nervous system, 151
meningitis by *Escherichia coli*, 165
meningitis by gram-negative bacilli, 166
Torticollis, 68
Toxic delirium, drug-induced, 190
Toxoplasmosis, 172, 173
Tranquilizers
contraindication in hepatic encephalopathy, 117
in treatment of postherpetic neuralgias, 112
Transaminases, serum glutamic
oxalacetic (SGOT), 37, 43, 46, 63, 135
pyruvic (SGPT), 37, 43, 46, 135
Tremor, essential, 70
Triamcinolone, and neuromuscular syndromes, 193
Tricyclic antidepressants, toxic delirium by, 190
Trigeminal neuralgia, 111
Trihexyphenidyl, in treatment of Parkinson's disease, 57
Trimethadione (TMO)
as antiepileptic drug, 46, 47
metabolized to dimethadione (DMO), 46
Trimethoprim, 151, 173
Trimethoprim-sulfamethoxazole, in treatment of meningitis associated with toxoplasmosis, 173

Trivastal (piribedil), in treatment of
Parkinson's disease, 56, 63, 65
Trypanosomiasis, 172, 173
Tryptophan, metabolism to nicotinic
acid (niacin) of, 128
Tuberculous meningitis, 169–170
Tularemia, 185
Tyramine-rich food, 192

Vaccines and brain syndromes, 192
Valproate, as antiepileptic drug,
35–38, 44–47
administration and blood levels, 36
formulation and indications, 35
in pregnancy, 37–38
interactions, 36–37
mechanism of action, 35
myoclonic seizures, 47
names (chemical and proprietary),
35
partial complex (temporal lobe)
seizures, 45
pharmacokinetic parameters,
35–36
relevant side effects, 37
tonic-clonic seizures (primary or
secondary grand mal), 44
Vancomycin, in treatment of
infections of the central nervous
system, 152
meningitis by *Staphylococcus*, 161,
164
Vidarabine (adenine arabinoside,
ARA-A), in treatment of encephalitis by *Herpes simplex*,
156, 184

Vincristine, to support nitrosoureas in
treatment of malignant
gliomas, 133–135
Viral meningitis, 169
suspected, 175
Vitamin
A, and encephalopathy, 192
cyanocobalamin (vitamin B-12),
128
deficiency, 129–130
D, 27, 32
deficiencies, 127–131, 127*t*
folic acid, 49
deficiency, 131
in treatment of
alcoholic peripheral neuropathy,
122–123
diabetic peripheral neuropathy,
121, 122
K
in treatment of transient cerebral
ischemic attack, 80–81
to reduce neonatal bleeding and
clotting defects, 49
niacin (nicotinic acid), deficiency
of, 128
pyridoxine (vitamin B-6), 155, 173
deficiency, 131, 191
thiamine, deficiency of, 129

Warfarin sodium. *See* coumarin
Water intoxication, 116
Wernicke's syndrome and thiamine
deficiency, 129
Wilson's disease (hepatolenticular
degeneration), 65–66